RUNNING
IN
REAL LIFE

Jenna Pogue

Trainer icon by Rizky Mardika on www.iconscout.com

First printing: 2023
Published by SBR Publishing
ISBN: 978-1-3999-4620-9

British Cataloguing Publication Data:
A catalogue record of this book is available from The British Library.

Also available for Kindle.

Contents

Introduction

Let me start with a bold statement: I decided to write a running book on a whim!

Yes, it's true. A whim, and that should begin to set the tone of this book for you. I'm not a professional writer. I'm not even a particularly good runner. I do, however, enjoy both activities in an entirely average way and I needed something to occupy my days during the COVID-19 pandemic.

During that time, my friend Penny was writing a book about wild swimming and it sounded like a fun process, so I figured, "Hey, what's the worst that could happen?"

As it turns out, I'm not Dr Pepper (if you don't know, look it up) and there were many times throughout the writing process when I regretted my sudden diversion from doing nothing with my life to writing a running book.

Although starting the book was decided on a whim, I had been threatening for a few years to put my own and my friend's running shenanigans down in print and although I had an abstract notion of what that book might be like, I never really committed to actually writing it.

Yet fast forward 24 months and here it is, all

finished – my book about running in real life*.

So, what exactly happened in those 24 months from when I decided to write a book to it actually becoming this book that you are reading now? Well, in the briefest sense, I had to try and recall everything I've ever known, heard, read, seen, or thought about running and then describe it in approximately 70,000 words that hopefully made sense to other human beings, especially runners or aspiring runners.

Despite being, at best, a mediocre runner I absolutely love it; I consider it 'my thing' and I take quite a lot of pride in calling myself a runner. I get a glowing sense of 'smug-face' when I tell other people about the running I've done (whether they asked to hear about it or not).

I imagine you feel the same way that I do about running, otherwise why would you buy a running book? Well yes, OK, I suppose you might have received a copy from your colleague Sharon in the office Secret Santa (thanks, Sharon!) but most likely you have it by choice (thanks, reader!), which means you are already a runner or you are considering becoming one in the near future. In both cases, you might be wondering what *Running in Real Life* has to offer you.

Let me answer that honestly: potentially, nothing.

---

*At the time of writing this line, the book is/was nowhere near finished. I am/was just eternally optimistic! (Plus a little undecided about the correct tense to use when writing about something that had not happened at the time of writing but had happened by the time the reader read about it…)

As an experienced runner, you may already know everything in this book, in which case I'm hoping you just laugh along with it, nodding your head and thinking: "Yep, that happened to me once."

If you are an aspiring runner, you might be completely horrified to hear what running can really be like and vow never to set foot in a pair of running shoes. If that turns out to be the case, at least you found out now, before you started losing toenails.

Running in Real Life is intended to be funny, light-hearted, down-to-earth and conversational. If you find it is not any of those things, there are two possible likelihoods: either it's a bad book or you have no sense of humour. We'll never know for sure which is correct, but I have my suspicions.

To avoid any confusion, here are a few things *Running in Real Life* is not:

- It is not a guide book or a 'how-to' on the art of running
- It is not an autobiography of my amazing personal journey through running (because I've had no such thing)
- It is not any one person's biography of their amazing running journey
- It is not an audiobook

To be fair, that last one should be obvious.

So, what exactly is *Running in Real Life*?

Well, it is a book. And it is about running – so I think I'm off to a good start. Essentially, it is a collection of anecdotes, stories and race reports all related to running and all of which I believe reflect running in its purest form. It is the story of how runners run in real life when it is not being glamorised for media or social media and when we're not pretending it's the perfect hobby all the time. Actually, sometimes running is kinda shit.

Sometimes you even shit yourself.

Some of the tales you are about to read are mine. Some were shared with me by my running friends, acquaintances, and random strangers off the internet. There's even plenty of input from my non-running friends and family who have a surprising amount of insight on running. Possibly because it's all they ever get to hear about.

I feel as if a metaphor might be a nice way to round off this introduction. I liken *Running in Real Life* to a table top at a jumble sale – it's got bits of everything. Running bric-a-brac, if you will. And, like bric-a-brac, most of it is tat, but there could be the odd gem if you look hard enough! I hope you find it.

And that's it in a nutshell. Which is what I'm led to believe a book introduction should be.

Read on at your leisure…

Chapter One
First Things First

I thought I would begin with a chapter on running 'firsts' – that is, the things runners find out straight away, the things that happen to us all and the lessons we learn, usually the hard way. I've also included the most basic things to note about me. Please don't think I'm entirely self-absorbed; I just thought I should explain what qualifies me (in the absolute loosest sense of the term!) to write a running book and why I wanted to do it.

I've been a runner for over eight† years now and for almost all of them I have been a member of Massey Ferguson Running Club in Coventry.

I've benefitted in many ways from being a runner and hitching my wagon to the running club. Physically would be the obvious one but I've also reaped the social, mental and emotional benefits, all of which I'll discuss more throughout the book, both from my own perspective and from others who have benefitted in the same way. Over the years, I've taken part in lots of fantastic races, countless training sessions and many social events that I remember

---

† Note to self: don't forget to change that number if it takes you years to finish the book. Also, don't forget to delete this note from the final edit or the readers will think you're an amateur.

through a bleary eye and, of course, the photographic evidence that exists on social media. I have also led training runs for the club, helped deliver our core strength sessions and I've been on the club's committee as joint social secretary with my sister-in-law Jo. I'll introduce Jo now as she is my most prolific partner in running crime. Actually, that's pretty much all the introduction she needs.

Most of the roles within the running club came about because I am easily led:

"Hey, Jenna, would you ever consider leading a run?"

"Oh go on then, you've twisted my arm with your incredibly persuasive question."

I'm not complaining, though, as all of this has given me plenty of time to experience the wonderful, heart-warming, positive benefits that running has to offer… but the only reason I feel I can write a running book of this nature is because I've also ventured to the dark side!

I was always torn about whether to call this book *The Dark Side of Running* but I worried that people would think it was some kind of *Star Wars* mash-up, fan fiction. I know even less about *Star Wars* than I know about running, so that would be a very disappointing book.

If you don't already know it, there exists a side to running that is only talked about within the inner circle. We have a little bit of a *Fight Club* situation going on when it comes to the rules, talking, and talking about the rules. I am generally a follower of rules and have a good moral compass but at the same time I am also an avid talker, so I really don't think anyone who knows me will be surprised that I'm here, talking about running despite the potential *Fight Club* consequences. There is a running meme doing the rounds that really hits home for me. It suggests that if anyone were to kidnap me, they would promptly return me right back to my owners after a meagre two hours of listening to me talking about parkrun (more on parkrun later).

To the dark side of running then. It is sticky, sweaty, bloody, and full of crap. Literally! (Again, more on that later.) It is littered with bad language from potty-mouthed, angry, tired runners who don't want to hear "Nearly there!" another fucking time. It is often in poor taste (yes, you in the camel toe leggings, taking a sneaky photo of your mate peeing over a farmer's hedge). It has eye-watering moments (Simon Neale, I'm thinking of you and that time you collided with the bollard) and of course there are all the hang-your-head-in-shame experiences (anyone who has ever had to use a buff as toilet paper, I am obviously referring to you).

Crucially though, it's this dark side that most runners love the most.

If they are brave enough to admit it.

I certainly enjoy the less glamorous side of running and it's given me all the content I need for this book, so there's that!

On the day I sat down to write *Running in Real Life* – the day after my whim – I began by thinking about what could go wrong for a runner and made a list of possible topics. I came up with 24 things just from my own experience alone. That's 24 potential opportunities for runners to embarrass and shame themselves like I had done in the past. At this point, I realised I could easily turn this book into a memoir and write about each topic from my perspective. I decided not to do that, for mostly selfish reasons (in other words, I don't want to embarrass myself too much!), and instead I invited runners from my club and further afield to submit their own stories and anecdotes alongside mine. Some are funny and some are really funny but I think most will be relatable to you and I'm fairly certain all of them demonstrate that running – 'real' running! – has a human side. Hence why I went with the title *Running in Real Life*.

Well, that and to avoid any *Star Wars*-based confusion.

My own running journey began in 2014 when I literally woke up one day and thought, "I'm going to start running today." Clearly I've always been prone to whims! I put on some rubbish old trainers that were too small, very old and not meant for running. I ran a quarter of a mile in total, from my front door, out and back. Eight years later, I still smile when I get to that eighth-of-a-mile turning point on my road.

That fateful day I was glowing red, sweating, gasping for air but at the same time I felt fantastic. I spent the last few metres up to my front door wondering who I should talk to about getting onto the Team GB Olympic squad. That, and I was mentally planning my social media post so everyone would know I had run. I didn't know much about running at that point but instinct told me it had to be shared somewhere for it to 'count'.

I shouldn't have gotten too carried away though… Six weeks later, I was on crutches. I had a semi-serious case of Achilles tendonitis caused by a trifecta of rookie mistakes:

1) a sudden increase of high impact activity;
2) running uphill (I always thought it was flat around where I live);
3) wearing poor quality shoes.

I quickly realised running is not always the perfect pastime those social media 'motivational' quotes would have you believe. You know the ones: there's a svelte runner in tiny pants, there's usually a sunset, occasionally there's a unicorn. They pontificate the virtues of running with words like 'posivitude' and 'believedness' and 'destinydom'.

By the way, it's really hard to make up fake motivational-sounding words to prove a point!

That initial injury cost me a lot of money to repair – I didn't know sports therapy existed prior to this – and has given me jip every so often, ever since.

I also quickly realised I am never going to be the toned and tanned runner/gazelle that graces the front cover of running magazines and books. Every time I go running I have to lug nearly 12 stones of middle-aged-woman body around with me. There's lots of wobbling and chafing. I console myself with a reminder that the standard of a superstar athlete can only be truly measured and appreciated because a mediocre runner like me also exists – there is no good runner unless there is a bad runner. I'm basically performing a service to the better runners out there. You're welcome, Eliud! I got you!

One of the first things we have to face as a runner is the myriad of myths.

Long before my whim (the one to start running), when all the people around me seemed to be getting into running and parkrun was making headlines, it felt like everything was pointing me towards taking up running as well.

However, I had a list of firmly held myths and anxieties on standby and I planned to use every one of them to get me out of running whenever someone suggested I join in with the nation's new favourite pastime.

They weren't going to suck me in! I was far too shrewd for that...

From my discussions with other runners it seems that most of us felt the same when we first ventured into the world of running. We all had various assumptions that were holding us back/we were using to delay the inevitable. These were mine:

- I'm too slow
- I'm too old (I was an ancient 29 at the time I

started running.)

- Running clubs are just for professionals (Even I actually LOL at this one now, knowing what I know!)
- Runners are elitist and won't accept me
- Everyone will hate me
- I can't go running if I don't have the right kit
- It'll be all men and I'll have nothing in common with them
- I'll be stuck at the back of every run
- Running is bad for my knees
- I'll hurt myself
- I'm not fit enough to start running
- Membership to a running club is too expensive (As it turns out, joining the club was the cheapest part. £33 per year, bargain!)

Most of my running friends also thought you had to be young, slender, fast and fit to run or join a running club. We all know now that it's simply not true and most local running clubs accept all sorts of level of runner; any size, any ability, any age, any gender, any hair colour and so on. I say 'most' because I know of one that actively turns away slower runners but that's definitely not the norm. This particular club is a bit of a breeding zoo for super-fast runners so I can understand them not wanting to water down their stock with an average Joe like me!

When Lisa, an accomplished ultra-runner (a runner who completes distances longer than the official 26.2-mile marathon distance), first got into running, she was under the impression that walking or resting during a race was not allowed. In fact, many of the runners I spoke to when writing this book expressed to me that they initially thought you would be disqualified for walking in a race. Lisa also thought it would be OK to run in Converse pumps when she first started out!

To be fair, Lisa can be forgiven for that one. Although not ideal for most runners, I've definitely been lapped at my local parkrun by an elderly gentleman wearing pumps. When Stuart, my significant other, first started at parkrun, he was lapped regularly by a man running in jeans.

You might be expecting me to share some helpful advice about how I overcame my fears and dispelled those myths but really my unconscious brain did all the hard work. It was very much the case that one day I believed my ankles were too puffy to be a runner and the next day I woke up and said, "OK, I'm going for a run today." Not particularly helpful if you are an aspiring runner hoping I'd allay some of your fears, but that is how it happened for me.

If pressed, I would say perhaps I was more influenced than I realised by those around me who had taken up running, many of whom I was really surprised by. My very unfit friends were running. My formerly lazy friends were running. Stuart, the aforementioned significant other, was running – and he was the epitome of laziness. My girlfriends were running, so obviously women were allowed to run and join running clubs. How naïve I'd been!

On my first day of running, I decided that if I enjoyed it, I would run alone for a while and get up to a certain level of 'expertise' before joining my local running club. That didn't quite go to plan as I was so buzzing after that first quarter-of-a-mile run that I went straight online and signed up to Massey's. I immediately started telling everyone who would listen that I was a runner and running was just a way of life for me now!

After joining the running club, I then decided I should still try to get up to some semblance of 'expertise' before joining one of their Wednesday night training sessions. Unfortunately, as I mentioned, I found myself in a pair of really rubbish trainers and injured!

By Christmas 2014 the Achilles tendonitis had healed, thanks to my awesome sports therapist, Charlotte. (Do other runners count their sports therapists amongst friends now too?) I was a proud member of a running club but I had yet to run with them. Apparently, I had talked enough about running though, even through an injury, that under the tree on Christmas morning was a printout giving me membership to a coveted spot on Massey's award-winning New Year's RaceFit course. RaceFit is a 45-minute session of core, mobility, strength, conditioning and balance workouts followed by a short run or running drills. It's all the things a good runner is supposed to do on a regular basis. I am a prolific attendee to this day, committing to at least one session every 6-8 weeks!

This particular Christmas gift, that I never knew I wanted, was from Stuart. I've mentioned him three times now so let me introduce him in a little more detail, as he does come up somewhat regularly throughout the book.

Stuart:

- is a runner and triathlete
- is tall
- is bald
- has an untamed beard that he thinks is 'hipster' but it's really just scruffy (like when people describe tatty furniture as 'shabby chic' when it's actually just old and broken)

And that's pretty much all there is to know!

Stuart has been running far longer than I have and I recall him coming back from roughly his fifth parkrun, long before I even considered running myself, muttering something about "I've beaten my parkrun PB three weeks in a row now." I had no clue what PB meant at that point but despite my ignorance, I figured out that whatever had happened was a good thing because he was smiling, which doesn't often happen with Stuart.

PB, for the record, means Personal Best. In other countries you might refer to a PR – a personal record. In either case, it means beating your previously held time in a certain race or distance.

Upon his declaration, I responded with a fairly lacklustre "That's nice," and carried on cleaning the windows. I really didn't care about running or PBs. At that point. The following Saturday I was laid up in bed with the flu, barely able to move, when my phone rang at around 9:25. It was Stuart, insisting that I get in the car immediately and bring his forgotten parkrun barcode to him because he had gotten another PB and it had to be recorded on his parkrun records to count.

My own parkrun PB lies unbeaten for over three years now. If anything, I'm getting further away from it, but I do have some vague recollection of that burning desire to knock seconds off my time, so I have forgiven him his demands that snotty morning.

In the build-up to that same Christmas, as a fully-fledged member of Massey Ferguson Running Club who had not yet run in a training session, race, or even set foot inside the clubhouse, I decided I would go to their Christmas party anyway. It seemed from the invite really quite upmarket. It was at a local golf club; it was black tie and the three-course dinner came with wine. A real classy do!

It did cross my mind whether it would be a bunch of running wankers who would only accept me following successful completion of a lengthy running-related hazing.

How wrong I was!

I decided early on not to include photos in this book – I never knew if I'd be publishing it myself and paying out of my own pocket, so frivolous extras like glossy pages and colour printing were the first things to go. I regret this now, as the best way to explain to you how wrong I was about the running club runners would be to show you the photos from that Christmas party! Photos that I know some runners wish would disappear forever. But they won't; they're still on my old phone. I just need to charge it up…

In lieu of photos, I'll try and paint you some word pictures...

- A female runner is draped over a table strewn with empty glasses, swigging from a bottle of wine and clutching her own boob
- A female runner is licking the cheek of a drunken runner who is passed out on another table covered with empty wine glasses
- A selfie taken in the toilet; the shot is filled with a close up of this runner's bra (this was taken when she stole my phone – a party trick that went on to become a running club party tradition)
- A male runner plants a wet kiss on the bald head of a fellow runner. The bald guy is drunkenly grinning, a dribble of saliva running down his chin
- A female runner, the ladies' captain, is squatting low on the dancefloor in a floor-length formal ball gown. She is fist-bumping the air as she twerks
- A male runner slumps drunkenly on a dining room chair, his head lolling, oblivious to the female runner straddling him and making rodeo gestures with her arm

I hope that's enough to give you a taste of why I was so wrong! These were not running wankers; these were party animals.

I was recently speaking to the fabulous Wendy, a long-time runner with the club, who summed it up perfectly: "You might think we are a running club with a drink problem, but we are actually a drinking club with a running problem."

This is something I've witnessed over and over again throughout my years in a running club. Real runners like to run hard but they like to party harder. It's like Spring Break every weekend in our club. "Runs out, guns out!" is one of our mottos. Well, that and "Don't be shit."

The hashtag #isurvivedfairytaleofnewyork was invented following a Christmas party in 2019 where numerous local running clubs came together to celebrate and the ensuing chaos when the DJ played The Pogues left some runners very bruised!

And shoeless!

And soaked in spilled whisky!

Despite their drunken shenanigans, I do have to give a bit of a serious shout-out to my running club – many of the stories in this book came from them. Or were caused by them!

The club, founded in 1977 at the Massey Ferguson tractor factory, has a long history in Coventry. As well as their party-animal reputation, Massey Runners are famed on the local running scene for being one of the friendliest clubs around, encouraging both faster and slower runners to co-exist. The club was formed on 21st November 1977 by a runner named Terry Lawson, who gathered together runners from the Massey Ferguson tractor company and formed a team to race against other firms in the area. To enable the club to compete in an official capacity, it had to be registered and have its own running vest and colours. It was at this point our iconic red and white quarters came into existence, designed by Terry Brown and quite distinct in style to other running vests at the time, which were usually striped or blocks of colour. You can easily spot our runners on race days in their red and whites. The only trouble is you might confuse us with Watford Joggers, who also wear the distinctive red and white quarters! I've eagerly waved at many a Watford Jogger in a race before realising it's not a club mate but a random stranger. I'm told there's even a third club out there now rocking the same style, so we obviously started a trend with our club colours. If you do see someone donning red and white quarters in a race, give them a wave – there's a chance they could be one of my Massey mates!

As great as it is, Massey's is not rare; pretty much every city and town you can think of will have a running club or running community these days. The benefits of joining a running club, whether you're a new runner or you have a little more longevity, are fairly obvious – you get to spend time with like-minded people, for a start. You get their support, friendship, banter and even their empathy when it all goes wrong. The downside to being surrounded by so many other runners, however, is that they are all very encouraging. I admit this doesn't sound like a downside but when you have 100+ lovely runners all telling you "You can do it!" you very quickly find yourself signed up for races and distances that you never wanted to even consider.

Almost all new runners experience this and, spurred on by the love and support of your club mates, you will find yourself caught up in something I call The Running Exponential (I'm an avid fan of *The Big Bang Theory* and I like to give random life moments a scientific title!).

This particular premise goes like this:

Running Day 1: "I just want to be out in the fresh air and get a little bit fitter. I don't want to run fast or run too far. I don't want any pressure."

Running Day 28: "I might consider a 5k one day. I say might; we'll see. I don't want to limit myself but I just don't want to do too much and feel pressured."

The day after your first 5k: "That was good. I could probably do a 10k if I really wanted to but I'm not going to put any pressure on myself."

A few weeks later: "Woohoo, 10k in the bag!"

The day after your next 10k: "If I were to even consider possibly doing a half marathon one day, I know it would only be a slow one and I'd probably have to walk a lot of it, at the back. I do think I could just about manage the distance though, so I might see if there's a flat one nearby maybe. Perhaps next year.

Just to see if I can do it. It would be nice to know if I could. That'll be me done though; I'd never consider a marathon. That's going too far. Too much pressure."

Shortly after your first half marathon: "Well, I've trained 4 nights a week for a year, done 17 x 5km, 5 x 10km, 2 half marathons and I'm signed up for a full marathon next week. Do you want to sponsor me?"

And, just like that, you are no longer the newbie at the running club. You're the one doling out the clichés and platitudes to the new wave of runners, telling them they'll be running marathons before they know it. They will be adamant that it'll never happen, just like you were! Just like we all were!

I only know of one runner who vowed on day one never to run a marathon who has yet to break that promise, years into their running. Congratulations, beautiful Denise, you've done what the rest of us couldn't manage and stayed true to yourself!

For a select few runners, the dialogue above will continue into running ultra-distances. I have myself uttered the words "I might consider an ultra, one day" (after only ever doing one marathon) and there was a brief moment in time when I genuinely thought I could do one. I was caught up in the occasion of watching a friend of mine tackle the local ultra-event, A Coventry Way, which is a 40-mile circular route around the outskirts of Coventry.

After a fantastic start to their ultra-training, their final sessions were hindered by the COVID-19 pandemic and their race day was postponed. When restrictions eased somewhat and my friend finally came to race, their grit and determination was even more inspiring and a small, socially distanced group of club members turned out to greet them mile after mile with cheers, hugs, and beers. They looked tired but they kept going, so it certainly didn't seem impossible to run 40 miles. As they knocked back a celebratory beer and fist-bumped supporters at the end, I found myself thinking I could do the same.

What you forget as a spectator, though, and what I forgot on this particular occasion was that you only see the runner for a snapshot of the race. In those few passing seconds, they seem OK, they can utter a few words or a wave, they say no to a jelly baby – so they must have energy left, right? However, what you don't see are the long miles up to that moment or the long miles after they pass you. It's hard to fully grasp the extent of an ultra-journey unless you are on it, as the reality of the distance becomes a bit blurry when you are just a spectator. I last saw my friend at mile 35; they were smiling and, crucially, still upright and moving forward. An ultra-race definitely seemed doable to me and I vowed to complete A Coventry Way one day. It's a vow I still cling on to.

As I write this, I realise that earlier today I walked up the stairs whilst talking on the phone and I couldn't catch my breath at the top. But a 40-mile ultra-run? Yep, sign me up!

There's another kind of 'ultra' runner that you might find yourself morphing into. It's not one who covers the ultra-distance in one go but the kind who goes to ultra-lengths to complete as many marathons as possible. There's an institution known as the 100 Marathon Club which exists to promote marathon running and celebrate the achievements of people who run 100 or more marathons. A proud member, and indeed founding member, of the 100 Marathon Club is my running friend Dave Phillips MBE, who is actually now carving out a path in the Over 500 Marathon Club. I have done one marathon (which was actually as part of Dave's team running for The Brain and Spine Foundation) and the training took up so much of my time, energy and emotional capacity that I can't fathom what it takes to run 500 of the bloody things! Over the years, Dave and his teams have raised more than £140,000 for charity and at the 2017 London Marathon, together with our friend Kelvin, we raised £9,000 running as Team Phillips. Dave has been featured in another running book by author Helen Summer, a book named *Running Crazy,* and that's the most perfect title if ever there was one for the likes of this particular Dave. I know a lot of running Daves – they're not all crazy! Just the ones who like to run 500 marathons. (Dave is on number 501 but has also somehow found the time and energy to have done 362 half marathons as well!)

We may not all reach the heady heights of 500 marathons, but most runners will have at least a first race at some point. Even if you initially planned to just run around your estate, the running community is fairly cult-ish and, one way or another, you will find yourself sucked in! My first race was a 5k in March. On an airfield. Needless to say, it was freezing bloody cold. It seemed like a huge challenge at that time and my main concern was that I would do something 'wrong' – that I would make a running faux pas.

I asked Stuart bizarre questions like "How will I know where to stand?" and "How will I know when to start?" and "Will other people think I'm a real runner and try to talk to me about running?" It was like I was new to being human, not just new to running!

I felt a conflict. I didn't want people to think I was a real runner and ask me a question I couldn't answer but I also didn't want them to think I was a newbie. I decided that, to avoid looking too inexperienced, I would not overdress. Layers, coats and hats all seemed like something inexperienced runners would need, so I ran in just my club vest and a pair of fairly light leggings. I mentioned it was March, didn't I? On an airfield? If you look at the race photos, I am a nice cool shade of blue.

I actually don't remember feeling cold though – I think I had too much fun. However, looking back at those photos, I now realise all my fellow club runners were dressed in what made them comfortable – base layers, caps and gloves. I'd worried too much about whether I looked the part and actually caused what I was trying to avoid: looking like I didn't know what I was doing. Even to this day, some of my fellow racers laugh at me for turning up in such a skimpy outfit on one of the coldest days of the year.

Shortly after I completed the race, I went to the merch stand to buy one of the race T-shirts. At this race, T-shirts were not included in the entry fee as they were a little more customised than normal and thus had to be purchased. The T-shirt had all the participants' names printed on the back along with the race they had run that day. I thought it'd be a nice memento of my first ever 5k… except there had been a mistake by the organiser and some participant names were duplicated. If you read the T-shirt closely you will be led to believe I ran both the 5k and the marathon that day – quite a feat for a new runner!

The running bug got me that day and less than eight months later I was on the start line for my first half marathon.

In a book about running in real life, I wanted to make sure I captured stories told in the words of runners themselves. At the end of each main chapter, I have included a race report written by a running friend of mine – except this first one, which was written by me about that very first half marathon. Some of the race reports are related to the chapter, some are a tenuous link to the chapter and, where I ran out of ideas, some are entirely unrelated to the chapter they are attached to. Oh and some of them are contributed by entirely better writers than I am!

Race Report
Jenna's Las Vegas Half Marathon

"Good job, Las Vegas, you're awesome!" said in a phony American accent became the motto of our running club trip to Las Vegas in November 2015 for the Rock and Roll Marathon Series.

To set the scene for this race report, imagine the following movies all at once: *The Hangover*, *Ocean's Eleven* and *Run Fatboy Run*. Now, with that in mind, read on to find out what happened when they let the dogs out. (If you know, you know!)

What do you call 12 runners in Las Vegas?

"Fucking idiots."

According to one occupant of a New York New York hotel 'elevator' in which a bunch of us were indeed acting like fucking idiots. The Rock and Roll Las Vegas Expo slogan was "You're kind of a big deal" and we had watched *The Hangover* one too many times while preparing for the trip, so we were living our best lives, our attitudes verging on cocky. We didn't do much for the reputation of the polite, unassuming British people!

The lift incident involved the much-aggrieved American standing quietly waiting to arrive at her floor with our party loudly repeating "Toodalooo motherfuckeeeeer!" every time the lift door slowly closed (if you've watched *The Hangover*, you'll know where that came from).

The banter had actually started on the plane. It was filled with mostly runners heading to the race and ophthalmologists heading to their annual eye conference. Oh, and stag dos. You could tell the cabin crew really hated this particular flight, what with the runners loudly discussing running, the ophthalmologists explaining the innate workings of the eyeball and the pissed-up stags chanting "We love you Burnley, we do." (This trip also resembled *The Inbetweeners Movie* in many ways, just with fewer 50-euro fines, thankfully.)

A meagre 20 minutes after landing, we'd already lost a runner! You'll know from most race days that when you can't find a runner, you check the loo. However, on this occasion Mylénè was actually locked inside the blacked-out limousine we had hired to take us to the hotel. She probably wouldn't have been in there too long normally but, being the best tourists we could be, we each wanted to take our own selfie with the limousine, followed by a group photo with the limousine, followed by a group photo holding our running club flag in front of the limousine, followed by just the half-marathoners on their own in front of the limousine, then the marathoners in front of the limousine. I lost track of how long Mylénè was actually locked inside!

I hadn't ever intended to run the Las Vegas Half Marathon – I didn't even know it existed – but after a post-training social, I was 'encouraged' (AKA persuaded, forced, manipulated) by my running friends into signing up for the 10k race. Was it ridiculous to fly 6,000 miles on an 11-hour flight for a 10k race? Yes, but I was going to do it anyway – they'd already added me to the Vegas Baby WhatsApp group!

Back at home, logging on to the website, I realised just how ridiculous it was and so I did the only sensible thing and signed up for the half marathon instead! At this point, I had never imagined running a half marathon and was still enjoying my new-found love of 10ks. Stuart couldn't justify going all the way to Las Vegas for a half marathon so I said it was OK for him to stay at home. As it turns out, he didn't want to cook for himself for a week so instead he went the whole hog and signed up for the full marathon!

Descending on Las Vegas on Thursday evening, we planned to hit up a local line dance bar and had bought the obligatory pink feather cowgirl hats before leaving the UK. However, after spending too much time, and pissing away our beer money, at the expo (I do still use my $30 phone holder actually), we slunk back to our rooms, exhausted.

The next morning we headed out early to sightsee and tick off some of our normal pre-race customs. Stuart, for example, was keen to get a massage to get the blood flowing and loosen off his legs ahead of Sunday. Try as he might though, he could not find anywhere offering massage of the bio-mechanical, musculoskeletal kind. Had he wanted the other kind of massage – the kind that ends rather more happily than a sports massage – all he would have had to do was stand still on the street for 20 seconds and wait for a 'business' card to be thrust into his hand.

Over the next few days we walked miles, visiting all the famous hotels, giving no thought to the distances we would run at the weekend. Many of the group also ate three times a day at our hotel restaurant, Chin Chin – a multi-cultural-inspired buffet that served up larger-than-life pancakes (the size of your head, seriously!), wings, ribs, mac and cheese, pizzas, Peking duck… I could go on but I'm sure everyone has been to an all-you-can-eat buffet. Just multiply what you know by 10 and you'll understand what a Vegas one consists of.

Our pre-race prep was certainly not what the how-to books suggest doing in the days building up to a race but we are real runners and this was Las Vegas. It cost us thousands to get there to do the race of a lifetime, but that wasn't going to stop us stuffing our faces, drinking beer and dancing in the street with showgirls! As the races are run at night to fully experience the magnificence of the Vegas Strip, Chin Chin was also the place many of us chose to eat breakfast and lunch on race day. I was on my fourth plate of mixed starters just three hours before the gun went off. They say not to try anything new on race day but I figured a lunch of lime jello (jelly) ribs and corn bread was worth any mid-race side-effects.

My first real understanding of how far 13.1 miles is had come the night before race day. We took the Las

Vegas monorail from our hotel, which was near the start line, to the Stratosphere hotel (now known as The Strat), which was close to the turnaround point for the half marathon. As the monorail pulled into the station, I burst into tears realising that if it seemed to take a bloody long time in a moving vehicle, how on earth was I going to manage it on foot tomorrow?

Back in the room a few hours later and still slightly sobbing, I prepared my first ever flat-lay. A flat-lay is when you lay out all your race-day running kit to ensure you have everything you need. It took me quite a while to prepare since I already knew that, more importantly than ensuring you have everything you need for the race, the flat-lay needs to look good in the Facebook post.

As many of you will understand, I was bricking it when I woke up the following morning. Whereas most races start early, Las Vegas races start around 4pm once the sun is setting, which meant I had plenty of time for the nerves to ramp up and also explains why I ended up at Chin Chin for my pre-race meals.

Eventually, after much waiting around it was time for our motley crew to head to the start line. As agreed, we were all going to run our own race so I joined my start corral alone. Well, not alone exactly, as the event attracts numbers in the tens of thousands, but alone from my club mates. After lots of shuffling in the corral, and a few emotional tears when it dawned on me what I was about to do, I finally crossed the start line at 5:15. Unexpectedly, it was raining for the first 5k and there were strong winds throughout (reportedly over 30mph) but it was easy to ignore the weather and become distracted by the noise and lights of Las Vegas. The route was flat and virtually a straight line out-and-back along the strip. There was such an exuberant atmosphere, I spent the whole race whooping and cheering, high-fiving spectators, touching hand-made posters for 'instant power' and singing along with the bands and DJs en route. The entire course was filled with neon and noise and took runners past everything that epitomises Las Vegas: the sign, the Bellagio fountains, Caesar's Palace (Caesar did not live there, by the way) and all the incredible hotels and sights and sounds. I was particularly lucky that the Mirage volcano erupted in glorious fashion just as I ran past.

For 7.5 miles, I ran at my most conservative pace, mostly due to my new-runner fear of collapsing, tripping, or injuring myself. However, at mile 8, I threw caution to the 30mph wind and sped up to a pace a little more challenging for me. Nothing bad happened, so I carried on. At 10 miles I saw four of the Massey girls in the distance, so I decided to sprint a little to catch them up – they were further away than I thought by the time I'd weaved in and out of the other runners (and walkers. This race attracts a strong walking crowd.) and I do wonder now if other runners thought I was a bit weird, breaking into a sprint with over 3 miles to go!

Heading into the last 5k, I had to do a lot more

weaving but as the route (which had taken us very briefly onto the darker, duller streets) turned back onto the glowing Las Vegas strip, I just kept reminding myself of that classic runner's mantra: "Only a parkrun to go" – although to be honest, I was actually starting to feel a little gutted that it would soon be over.

Finally, to a wall of sound, I crossed the finish line and collected my medal: an oversized, spinning, glow-in-the-dark slot machine! It was Vegas, after all, so it was bound to be brash! And I love it; to this day it is still one of my favourite medals I've ever earned and shoved in a box.

Chapter Two
Life As We Know It

I had always thought that running was a simple and inexpensive sport. Long before I knew anything about running. Long, long, before! Right now, I'm broke having just spent £135 on a pair of new Altras (running shoes) because I've gone off the pale blue of my barely worn Provision 5s and they've just released a really nice green, pink and orange colourway in the Provision 6s.

I also bought two new pairs of running leggings yesterday because "Oooh, I don't have any purple ones yet!"

I do have a couple of running friends who fight tirelessly to keep their running simple and inexpensive. They can be truly believed when they say they only run for the joy of it and that they have no real clue how far or fast they've run. Their only joy in running comes from actually running and the feelings it stirs up inside them. Naturally, they are far more noble and pure than those of us who just do it for the bragging rights and to bask in the glory of PBs. Who out of the rest of us doesn't love to go on Facebook after a race and see lots of red dots appear, each one informing us how amazing and inspirational we are?

Of the purists, I know two. Out of the hundreds of runners that I know. Just two.

As I write, I wonder if it could be quite a nice way to live as a runner and I consider whether I can try to emulate their pure passion during my own training later tonight. Maybe I won't take my watch?

I at once feel a sense of panic at the thought of turning up to tonight's session without a running watch because as we all know, if it's not on Strava it doesn't count. I'm editing this chapter shortly after the sad passing of Queen Elizabeth II and I heard that someone had even Strava'd their 5-mile journey through the lying in state queue.

Aside from not caring about Strava, I bet the few running purists out there also never check themselves out in a shop window as they run past. Whereas I, the narcissist runner, always enjoy a good, wide shop window on a run. I like to see if I look 'good'. If I look like a 'real' runner.

Spoiler alert!

I don't look good.

I look like a haggis, if a haggis could run!

I know what you are thinking: surely I am not vain enough to covet the perfect shop-window reflection or the perfect race photo that makes me look like an amazing runner, even though I claim not to care?

We've all heard words to the effect of "It doesn't matter what you look like, what's important is how you perform," yet often the first thing we do post-run is share our running selfies. If running is all about performance and not image, why do brands keep bringing out FAB-U-LOUS ranges of colourful, stylish kit and why did I just buy two new pairs of purple leggings? Whilst I was shopping, I saw a great pair of leopard print and mesh leggings. I'm not sure exactly how leopard print contributes to running performance but they were £15 more expensive than the plain black pair despite boasting the same technical qualities – reduced chafing, moisture management and a tiny pocket suitable for holding absolutely nothing.

So I'll just come out and say it and then, if you feel comfortable and in a safe space, you can follow my lead:

"I wish I looked good as a runner."

I have an image of what a 'perfect' runner looks like… toned, tanned, athletic, tall, battle-braided hair, £100 designer leggings. We have a handful of these runners in our running club and I have lovingly dubbed them The Beautiful People.

Sadly, it is a pipe dream for me. If I stand directly beside one of The Beautiful People you will notice that I am squishy, pale, short, scruffy, and wearing £9.99 see-through leggings (it's OK because I wear knickers!). But it shouldn't and doesn't matter. If you run, you're a runner. And that's the be all and end all! Although I'm not saying that if a genie in a lamp granted me the chance to become one of The Beautiful People tomorrow, I wouldn't snap his tiny hand off.

I recently saw a running meme posted by an 'influencer' in which they said: "If you still look cute after your run, you didn't run hard enough." Now,

I'm not sure who that bit of influencing is aimed at but let me tell you, it's not me! I don't even look cute before my run, let alone after. If you look at my pre-run prep checklist you'll come to realise why I begin a run already looking like a sweaty, sticky, flammable mess, only for it to get worse once any actual running begins. This is how my pre-run routine usually goes:

- Apply sports tape to broken bits (currently toes, forefoot, heel, ankle, soleus)
- Apply a layer of sunblock (I burn watching *Home and Away*, so a run in the actual sun is risky)
- Waft on a can of bug spray (they'll still swarm me but maybe only half will take a bite?)
- Apply a thick mist of hairspray (my hair is a mess before you add in sweat and sunblock)
- Slick on a layer of ibuprofen gel to anywhere not already covered in sports tape
- Down a cocktail of paracetamol, anti-histamines, and jelly babies
- Have four wees (minimum)
- Change kit because it's too hot/cold outside
- Change kit again because it's actually not too hot/cold outside
- Change back into original kit because now I've overthought it
- Tighten shoelaces
- Loosen shoelaces
- Change shoes altogether
- Relearn how to use my watch (the watch I've

39

had for four years)
- Look for the small key that fits into my tiny pocket
- Realise that, inexplicably, the small key is not where I left it after my last run

All that for a 5k training run!

When I told my friends about this list, the fabulous Cathy reminded me: "You forgot to take three Imodium." My other friend Super Dave (he runs extreme ultra races, hence the name) chipped in with, "I don't do any of that," and that was not surprising to me as Dave is one of the two runners I consider a purist. He just runs for running's sake and he covers impressive distances with it. There are no unnecessary bells or whistles on Super Dave's running; he just gets it done and enjoys it for what it is.

My post-run routine also does not lend itself to anything resembling 'cute'. For a start, I spend 20 minutes in the 'sweaty chair'…

The sweaty chair exists, next to a pile of cushions, throws and a bottle of Febreze, to allow Stuart and me to cool off and dry off, post-run, rather than traipsing through the house splashing sweat on the nicely painted walls. It provides a comfy spot from which to upload our Garmin and Strava activities, followed by any Facebook and Instagram statuses, before once again going back to Strava to check for immediate Kudos. We have to congratulate Stuart's dad, Arthur, on always being the first person to give Kudos on any activity – we think he sits refreshing Strava continuously as no sooner have we posted than we get notification of his admiration!

Only once the salt has started to harden on my face will I leave the 'sweaty chair' and go for a shower. Despite 20 minutes having passed since I finished running, I will still be bright red when I get in the shower and I'll be even redder when I get out. I then have to get the manky bag of peas out of the freezer to ice the swollen bits (usually it's the same bits that were taped up beforehand, sometimes it's new bits).

I don't know if any of you also have a manky bag of peas (wait, that's no longer true – Joy, I know you do!) but if you're anything like me, yours will be in dire need of replacement. They've been in and out of the freezer so many times, they must smell horrific.

After icing, I apply another layer of sticky ibuprofen gel.

This is a good time to point out that you should not copy my routine for the rehabilitation of your own injuries. I am not a doctor!

Next comes the really glamorous toe separators. These are gel contraptions that separate your toes (in case that isn't obvious) and they help keep my metatarsals separated, giving me some relief from the Morton's neuroma/bursitis complex I suffer with. Which was caused by cycling, not running, just in case any of my non-runner friends are reading this and starting to take pleasure in the fact that they always knew running wasn't good for me.

At this point, I flop down on the sofa (the good sofa,

not the sweaty chair) smelling of menthol, balancing manky peas in a chorizo-stained tea towel on my ankle with my toes separated by what looks like a dead jellyfish. I am red in the face, my hair is wet and tangled because there is no way I am adding to my temperature by pointing a hairdryer at my head, and I am in my post-run comfy pyjamas (which are the shorts from a Tesco men's loungewear set and a £1 Primark vest top). And I am still huffing a little because every run takes it out of me these days.

Cute?

I think not.

What I am, though, is smug.

Fast or slow, all runners (except the purists, because they are too noble) find themselves in a little place called Smug Town after a good race or run. We all enjoy that feeling of completing our race, smashing our goals, and sharing our joy on Instagram. In Smug Town, you get to wear the official uniform of 'smug pants' (AKA grey joggers) for the rest of race day and you can utter phrases such as "But I got a 10k PB today!" when your partner refuses to make you a cup of tea (no, it's not a big ask, but in my household you need a bargaining tool to get a cuppa). I fondly remember my early parkrun days when I would spend the whole day repeating "I ran 5k today" to get anything I wanted. Most Saturdays, I had a Chinese takeaway for dinner because "I ran 5k today."

When Jo completed her first parkrun, I had a Thornton's chocolate plaque iced with "I did

Parkrun." Yes, they did use a capital P and yes, it did sully the gesture in some people's eyes (more on that later if you don't know what I am referring to).

I always remember the assistant's face in Thornton's when I told her what I wanted iced on the plaque. It was mostly confusion. They mainly get requests for 'Happy Birthday' or 'Congratulations' and I think my unusual request threw her off guard for a second. I could see the cogs turning in her brain… this is for a runner… but it's a chocolate plaque… surely athletes don't eat chocolate?

Ha! What does she know!

I just Googled 'will run for chocolate' and found not only a running T-shirt with it printed on, but a mug, a notebook, a magnet, a chequebook and pen, a cuddly toy… OK, some of those I made up for effect, but you get my point… Runners love chocolate!

As much as runners love their sport, and chocolate, we also very much like finding various and novel ways to get out of a run. For many reasons – family, work, energy levels, the weather – sometimes the thought of a run is just the worst. It's something of a paradox as none of us would be without running, and any kind of enforced break through injury causes us turmoil, but still there are occasions when we simply don't want to go out.

If you need to back out of a run for shoddy, unathletic reasons, I've gathered all of the best 'excuses' and listed them below, giving you a set of pre-prepared, standard phrases to help you out in your time of need. They have all been quality assured by me personally and many have been through a second rigorous testing by various running friends when they have wanted to flake out on a run with me.

- It's pouring down
- I'm racing this weekend
- I raced last weekend
- My shoes are knackered
- My toenail's about to fall off
- I'm really badly injured
- My watch isn't charged
- Strava is down
- I can't get a signal on my Garmin
- I can't find my keys
- My kit is still wet
- I have the flu
- I'm going for a walk instead

If you are not the kind of runner who would make excuses and are shocked at the very thought, here is the same list for you, but with the truth behind each one in brackets so you can easily spot when your running friends are trying to pull a fast one:

- It's pouring down (there is a 5% chance of rain later tonight)
- I'm racing this weekend (the race is not for another five days)
- I raced last weekend (it was six days ago)
- My shoes are knackered (my shoe has a small

hole in the toe)

- My toenail's about to fall off (my toenail was mildly bruised a few weeks ago)
- I'm really badly injured (my legs are a bit sore from Yoga three days ago)
- My watch isn't charged (my watch has 60% battery)
- Strava is down (Strava is a bit slow but it's fine)
- I can't get a signal on my Garmin (I held my arm in the air for three seconds and nothing happened)
- I can't find my keys (I didn't look for my keys)
- My kit is still wet (all my other kit is perfectly dry)
- I have the flu (I coughed once this morning)
- I'm going for a walk instead (I am not going for a walk instead)

Have you realised yet what a fickle runner I am? One day running is the most important thing in the world to me and the next I'm pretending to be bed-ridden just to get out of a training run.

The one thing that I will never try to get out of though is talking about running!

If you ask any member of our family, they will tell you that Jo and I can turn any conversation into a running-specific one in 10 seconds or less:

"Do you want beef or lamb burgers for dinner tonight?"

"Oh, I had the best beef burger after a race once. I think it was Northbrook 10k. I had a great run that day; I really felt good on my legs, you know? I didn't quite get a PB but not all races are about that, are they? My best race ever was actually nowhere near my PB, I just really enjoyed the route and atmosphere that day."

"So? Beef or lamb?"

"Beef or lamb what?"

You can decide for yourself if this was a real conversation or not. And if Simon, Jo's husband, stabbed himself in the hand with a fork before he ever got an answer to what Jo wanted for dinner that night.

As runners, one of the things we have to get used to is that as soon as we express any kind of interest in the sport we will be getting running-related birthday and Christmas presents until the day we die. Yes, some of it is just what we want (usually only the case if we've asked for it) but most of it is complete crap. Well-intended and well-meaning crap. When you become a runner, your friends and family become experts at unearthing the most obscure running paraphernalia the internet has to offer. You are forever in danger of receiving a 'will run for chocolate' pencil case!

If it helps, here is a cut-out-and-keep of top tips that can be waved in front of your family and friends' noses shortly before any big gift-buy occasion.

How to buy gifts for the runner in your life

1. **Running socks make a great stocking filler.** Just remember to get your runner's correct size and preferred style. Some runners like a twin-skinned sock whilst others prefer a single layer. Always buy from a reputable running outlet – most runners are sock snobs and a pack of trainer socks from M&S that says they are 'ideal for running' will not usually cut it.

2. **Take care when buying other items of clothing.** Technical kit differs vastly in size between manufacturers and different items function in different ways. Reconsider buying kit if you haven't been given a very specific brand, size, and colour preference from your intended recipient. I tried on a running vest last week that looked great on the hanger and would have looked lovely wrapped up as a present; however, despite being my exact size it showed a great deal of side boob plus almost all front boob.

3. **Running books are an excellent choice.** They are 10/10 the best gift you could give to all the runners you know. They'll really enjoy one called *Running in Real Life*.

4. **I can't say it enough: running books, particularly the suggestion above, make excellent gifts.**

5. **Please be aware of running tat.** Your instinct may be to buy running-related mugs, keyrings, carriage clocks and so on but just because the word 'running' is on an item doesn't necessarily mean it will be either useful or ornamental to a runner. I was once given a runner-shaped toast cutter, which is ridiculous because everyone knows runners don't eat breakfast.

6. **Race entries can make a nice gift.** Just make sure you choose good races. With medals and T-shirts. Think destination races and you're along the right lines.

7. **A running watch is a pricey gift** but if you need to make up for something you've done wrong or want to secure yourself some brownie points to hold over your loved one in the future, consider items priced £200 and upwards.

Life as we know it then seems to be a battle of wills between a run-loving angel on one shoulder and an "I need an excuse to stay home" devil on the other. It is the joy of treating yourself to a fun pair of running leggings whilst forever being at risk of receiving an 'I ♥ RUNNING' coaster.

Above all, the life we lead as runners is a healthy, sociable one where we meet a lot of new people, most of whom are OK, and we challenge our bodies to achieve new things.

And we run, train and sign up to races, knowing we are part of a safe, fun, enjoyable (in a sadistic way) community where we can showcase our achievements and then celebrate with our friends and families afterwards. Races become a part of life for most runners; there's no more articulate way of describing it than "It's just what we do." So, I don't think anyone could have imagined that one day someone would target a world-renowned marathon in an act of terror. Sadly, that is what happened on April 15th, 2013 when two terrorists detonated home-made explosive devices within a short distance of the Boston Marathon finish line. The devices – pressure cookers – were packed with an explosive substance and shrapnel and detonated seconds apart, killing three and injuring hundreds. It's gut-wrenching to imagine the horror, fear and terror that those runners and spectators went through in the moment, in the aftermath and in the years to follow. Just normal everyday runners like ourselves, doing the one thing we all love to do without a second thought.

My incredible friend Kelsey was one of the runners taking part that day and she kindly shares her race report with us.

Race Report
Kelsey's Boston Marathon

"THERE IS NO BETTER FEELING THAN THIS!"

Surely there cannot be a better feeling than this?!

I had just crossed the finish line of the Boston Marathon, THE Boston Marathon, the oldest running marathon and one with huge prestige, and I had completed it! Although my legs felt like lead, I was shaking from fatigue, dehydration, and low blood sugar (I had no concept of actually fuelling for one of these things), I couldn't help thinking, "THERE IS NO BETTER FEELING THAN THIS!"

Fast forward one hour and the sentiment was completely different. The vast contrast in emotion couldn't be greater, truly from the highest of highs to the lowest of lows.

You see, the year was 2013. Ah, maybe you've clocked it now… 2013… Boston… Ooooh, THE BOMBING YEAR. Yes, I was one of over 23,000 runners privileged to earn a spot in the 2013 race. I got my qualifying time in May 2012 in my second ever marathon, but the first one I had actually trained for. I had been a bit rebellious in my first marathon, only signing up for the half and making the decision at the half-marathon/marathon junction to carry on with the marathon runners because why not?! I nearly qualified for Boston during that first impromptu marathon and that was all the fire I needed to actually train and qualify to run the infamous race.

I lived in Michigan at the time, so my training was mostly through the winter with really harsh weather; lots of snow and literally freezing my arse off! My motivation remained high; it was BOSTON I was training for, after all.

April finally rolled around and Patriot's Day was approaching fast. For those unfamiliar, Patriot's Day is not just the name of the Mark Wahlberg film but is in fact a holiday in Boston. It has something to do with commemorating the start of the Revolutionary War and all that jazz but for me, the significance was Marathon Monday. The 117th running of the Boston Marathon would take place on Monday 15th April 2013.

As I'm sure most fellow runners can appreciate, the night before any race is filled with excitement, anxiety, getting up to check you actually have your number and race pins, lots of self-doubt (26.2 miles is a fucking long way) and about five minutes of sleep. Boston is a point-to-point race, which means runners must get transportation to the start. This meant that although the start time of the race was a reasonable 10am, transportation was at 6am. It didn't really matter though; it's not like I was getting any shut eye.

My fellow marathoners and I filed onto school buses and were transported to the start… the start of the fucking Boston Marathon! Waiting to be called to the start corrals seemed like the longest wait ever, although that time was filled with visiting the port-a-potties around 10 times (fellow runners will understand!).

I still get an adrenaline surge just thinking about toeing the line. I was quite new to distance running but the significance of being one of the runners to make it to this point was not lost on me. The weather that year was great, a bit warm if anything but nothing too extreme. The wait was finally over... I had endured months of training and, potentially even worse, endured the nine-hour car journey with my parents to Boston. I'd made it through the sleepless night and here I was, getting ready to cross the blue-and-yellow-painted START.

The gun went off and so did my legs... perhaps a bit too quickly. I had been warned about not going out too fast, especially on this course, as the first mile is a net downhill. Containing my excitement, though, seemed near impossible and I just let my legs fly. I could not believe the atmosphere. Spectators were lining the course three or four rows deep in most places. It was like the people of Boston were having their own competition to see who could support the loudest.

I remember feeling a bit tired around mile 8 (a bit early to be hitting the wall) but the crowd was so immense my fatigue seemed to almost evaporate. Then around mile 11 I entered Wellesley College territory. I had never experienced anything like this. The college girls were out in full force, all with various signs stating, "Kiss me, I'm..." followed by some clever description. I witnessed a guy I had been running next to veer immediately right and stick his tongue down one of the girl's throats! I'm sure she appreciated the sweat-flavoured kiss. The atmosphere didn't let up from there either. The entire course was like running through a party; the energy was palpable and it truly made it hard to succumb to fatigue. Around mile 16 I saw my parents, who were spectating. Their cheers hit a bit deeper than the others and I felt an added boost.

There had been a lot of pre-race chat about Heartbreak Hill and what a soul destroyer it was, basically where marathon dreams went to die. Quite frankly, I must have repressed running up it and any difficulty it gave me. The rest of the race is a bit of a blur – that is, until I made that final turn onto Boylston Street.

HOLY SHIT! That's it, that's the actual finish line of the Boston Marathon! Just like that, my legs seemed to find an extra gear. I was doing it; with each step, I was getting closer and closer to crossing that oh so magical (there is actually a unicorn signifying it) finish!

I ran under the huge banner and saw the most beautiful painted word on any road surface I had ever seen: FINISH. I had done it! I fucking finished the Boston Marathon!!!

SURELY THERE COULDN'T BE A BETTER FEELING THAN THIS?!

The elation was short-lived, however, and that feeling will always be a bit tainted with the events that followed. I consider myself so lucky: so lucky to not have been harmed in the event, so lucky that I was able to reunite with my parents before the bombs went off, so lucky to have actually been able to cross that finish line and complete the race, and so lucky with how experiencing something so awful unexpectedly brought me the greatest gift and forever changed my life.

Immediately upon crossing the finish line I was donned with my medal and handed various food items and beverages. My poor shaking body could barely hold onto anything. I very gingerly made my way down the finishers' shoot, trying to keep hold of all the free shit I was being handed (even if I knew I would never consume a mint-flavoured protein bar, it was free, after all!). I kept walking, and walking, and OK, come on guys, I just ran bloody 26.2 miles, how much further do I have to walk?! Finally, I made it to the baggage claim where I could pick up the gear I had checked at the start line. More shit to carry now! Where are my parents? Not only did I want to see them and bask in their congratulations, but fuck, I really could use some help holding all this loot!

I was finally reunited with my two biggest supporters and it was such a tremendous feeling, and a literal weight off me as I dumped everything I had just accumulated into their arms. I told them I wanted to go back to the finish and watch some of the other runners achieve their dreams. They agreed it would be nice to support my fellow marathoners. Just as we were about to head back, a man asked me if I was in the queue. I looked a bit puzzled, so he elaborated: "Are you in the massage queue?" I had unknowingly been queuing (clearly born to be British) to get a post-race massage. I told the man I hadn't known there were massages and he explained that they were just beyond the doors in one of the nearby buildings. My legs did feel like absolute rubbish and although I felt sorry for anyone going near me to rub them, it sounded like a nice treat. I decided to remain in the queue and my parents and I could make our way to the finish afterwards…

I remember having to go down multiple sets of stairs once inside to get the massage. "This has to be a piss take!" I thought, as I was guided to go down the stairs backwards (clearly not some people's first marathon). While getting the massage, I remember hearing a loud noise. Nothing extreme or anything to cause alarm. "Maybe something upstairs fell over?" I thought, as I chatted away with the poor massage therapy student, who I hoped wasn't too repulsed by my salt-crusted skin and ripe odour. I graciously thanked the student, put my medal and shoes back on and hobbled upstairs.

As I opened the door to outside, I realised everything had changed. People were running with no sense of direction. Mothers were yelling out for their children. People were screaming, others crying. I kept hearing the word BOMB being thrown around. Others saying, "No, it must have been fireworks."

"Maybe it was thunder?" Then a few people had their phones out with news confirming that indeed there had been a bombing.

I couldn't quite get my mind around it. "Bombs? We're just a group of runners competing in a race. Why would there be bombs?" My parents looked equally confused. Luckily, I had been reunited with them immediately upon exiting the building from getting the massage. We kept looking in all directions, uncertain what to do.

We joined in with groups of confused runners and runners' families walking or jogging away from the finish area. There was talk that more bombs were hidden. I remember feeling sheer terror as I willed my tired body to walk as quickly as I could away from the area and back towards our hotel, which was a few miles away. I had my phone with me and I started receiving a massive influx of messages regarding the bombs. I don't think I realised the severity of the situation until I received a message from a runner friend from England, wondering about my wellbeing. "Shit, it's even hit news over in the UK?!" I compiled a quick Facebook post stating that my family and I were okay. Then they cut the phone lines, in case phones were used as a form of detonation.

The entire walk/jog back to the hotel I kept looking all around me, basically waiting for an explosion. I had never experienced such conflicting emotions in such a short amount of time. From sheer elation and joy to absolute terror and heartbreak.

Our hotel was a few miles from the finish line and next to a large hospital. The news speculated that maybe hospitals would be the next target for bombing. It was such an uneasy feeling; truly nowhere felt safe. We were told not to leave the hotel. I couldn't take my eyes off the news. I kept re-watching the footage from the explosions over and over.

"That could have been me."

I kept thinking about the man directing me into the massage queue and…

"What if I hadn't gotten a massage?"

The plan had been to go back to the finish line…

We spent a very uneasy night in the hotel. A few news crews from back in Michigan reached out to me. I truly didn't know how to process any of it. I'm not sure if I do to this day really.

Although it was truly a horrific day filled with tragedy, it did bring something, or rather someone, who would change my life in the best way possible. That runner friend from England that I mentioned reaching out to me when he heard about the bombings… Well, we're married now. Up until Boston, we had been following each other here and there on social media, becoming friends through a running app. We would comment now and again on each other's runs and what upcoming races we were going to participate in. He'd had to withdraw from the marathon he had been training for due to injury and he had wished me good luck for Boston; I was to run for both of us.

After going through such an extreme event, we started messaging a lot more. It took some months, but he eventually admitted that knowing I was at that race and having some moments of uncertainty about my well-being convinced him that perhaps there was something to pursue. Fast-forward to the present and we've been married for four years, I live in England now and we get to toe start lines together.

I went back and ran Boston again in 2017, with the best support crew: my parents and my 'runner friend from England'. As I crossed that finish line, I could only think…

THERE IS NO BETTER FEELING THAN THIS!

Chapter Three
The Clothes Maketh
The Runner

For most runners, there's nothing more frustrating than realising on race day that you have forgotten to pack something crucial in your kitbag. Something that you simply can't race without. Your heart sinks as it dawns on you that one of your trainers is 30 miles away at home, propping open the front door (true story!).

If you really think about it, though, there are only three things that should cause genuine panic should they be forgotten on race day:

- your number bib
- your timing chip
- your trainers

Anything else, you could probably still take part without, if you are really honest about it!

But we're runners and we're dramatic so we need every single item of kit and clothing to be available to us in exactly the same manner as it was during our training runs. As a group, we're not really very flexible, are we?

I've watched people get back into their car and leave a race just because they have forgotten their running watch. If that happened to me, I'd be crabby for a while, and of course when I considered leaving my watch at home on purpose, I got the shakes, but I like to think I would still run the race.

Having said that, I did once have a tantrum on a start line because I picked up the 'wrong' pair of trainers. I had grabbed my orange ones when I wanted my purple ones. It sounds silly, but it was a perfectly legitimate emotional response at the time; the orange ones had a little hole in the toe. No one could be expected to run a race wearing trainers with a hole in the toe.

Except Stuart. Every pair of trainers he owns seems to develop a small hole in the exact same spot after just a few runs. He must have one really long toe!

Anyway…

A friend of mine genuinely considered pulling out of a race because they left their spare socks on the hall table!

In those moments, as ridiculous as it sounds, it does feel like the end of the world. We are so programmed to not change anything on race day. If we don't record a run it means it won't count and if we don't coordinate our trainers with our vest we won't run as fast and if other runners somehow spot that our trainers have a teeny tiny hole in the toe, the entire race will have been pointless and our identity as a runner will be called into disrepute. I appreciate that it might be just me who is concerned about that last one.

So again, if you really think about it, sensibly,

perhaps through the eyes of a non-runner to gain some perspective, it really shouldn't matter if you forget a piece of objectively non-essential kit.

Let's say it's race day and you've forgotten your running watch. If you continue with this race, you will have no way of knowing your pace or distance and you will have no record of the run on your tracking app of choice (e.g. Strava, Garmin etc).

First, calm down. This is hypothetical. You are not at a race; you have not forgotten your watch. This is not a nightmare. You are sitting comfortably reading a running book. Relax.

So, anyway, you've forgotten your watch (breathe). Accept if you can, just for the next few sentences, that running a race actually has no dependency on wearing a running watch.

If you run a race from START to FINISH (which the race organisers will have clearly marked for you) then you have run the race from START to FINISH. That won't change either way with the absence or presence of a watch. During the run, you know you are running and after the run, you know you have run. The memory of running won't immediately be wiped from your mind when you cross the finish line just because you aren't wearing a watch. The watch literally has nothing to do with the run. They exist entirely independent of one another.

Yet for many (OK, probably most) of us, a forgotten watch would cast a dark cloud over race day and for some (perhaps more than would care to admit it), it would equal an abrupt end to race day. And in both cases, there'd be 12-24 subsequent hours of crankiness and mood swings.

A non-runner friend of mine once suggested to me that it's very irrational and childish to be cranky over not being able to race due to a forgotten piece of kit.

Don't worry, they are still alive. Although we are not friends anymore (for different reasons!).

"So you'd lose a few pounds on your race entry," they told me.

"So you wouldn't get a medal to throw in a drawer and never look at again," they chastised.

"So you wouldn't get another T-shirt to add to the 75 you already own."

By now, they'd made me feel really pathetic.

"I knooooooooooow!" I replied, like a moody teenager.

Of course I don't need another medal or T-shirt and yes, it wasn't hugely expensive in the grand scheme of things but you know what, my super-judgemental non-runner friend…?

…I was looking forward to running. I trained hard (or at least as far as you are concerned I trained hard!) and I'm entitled to feel cranky, thanks very much.

I know it shouldn't matter.

It absolutely does matter.

It is entirely my own fault if I forget something.

That is the worst part!

You might have been surprised when I mentioned a few paragraphs ago my friend who wanted to pull out of a race after forgetting her spare socks. You might be more surprised to find that she's not alone! At London Landmarks, close to the race start time, my wonderful friend Helen started patting herself down in a panic.

"I've forgotten my spare socks!" she gasped in horror.

We (me, Stuart and our friends Andrew and Hayley) were all silent. We weren't sure how to respond, none of us being accustomed to carrying spare socks. But Helen was accustomed to it and this was one of the kit items that she felt it necessary to have on standby during her race.

To you, spare socks might seem like an odd thing to pack into your pockets or running backpack, particularly for a road race, but I've actually found that many runners can't face the idea of stepping in a puddle or tearing a hole in their sock mid-run and then having to run feeling wet and uncomfortable. To these runners, a spare pair of socks balled up and stuffed somewhere safe, just in case, is a non-negotiable piece of race day kit that they can't run without.

I'm pretty sure that right now half of my readers are laughing at the idea that someone would even consider running with spare socks in a road half marathon. I'm equally as sure that the other half of my readers are shaking their heads and saying: "Wow, poor lady, I'd be beside myself if I forgot my spare socks on race day. What a terrible thing to happen to someone. Hope they're OK. Wonder if they want to DM me, hun?"

Don't worry, Helen was ultimately fine and ran a great race as always, thankfully with no need for spare socks. Which is a good job as it's not the kind of thing you want to borrow from another runner, is it? Asking for the loan of a safety pin... that's fine. Asking for the loan of spare socks, however, is quite something else.

Back in 2016, I had my own kit disaster – a genuinely disastrous one, not just me being dramatic over a forgotten pair of lucky race day earrings (another true story!).

Sidebar... Whether all these 'true stories' are mine or someone else's, I'm not going to confess!

In August of that year, I was taking part in Ironman Vichy 70.3 Relay in France.

Firstly, for anyone thinking I do Ironman triathlons, let me just clear something up...

...I don't!

My athletic friends do the big triathlons and I tag along to support them. I occasionally take part in some of the smaller ones myself, namely sprint triathlons where I can be finished and eating an ice-cream in a relatively short amount of time.

In this particular race, I was supporting my lovely friend Debbie by stepping in to cover the run element after she picked up an injury. A 70.3 is a half distance triathlon that includes a casual 1.2-mile swim, a 56-mile bike ride and a half marathon to finish.

Yes, all on the same day.

Yes, for fun.

Debbie took on the swim and the bike, which come first, in that order, so I had prepared myself for a morning of perusing the race village and expo, then cheering on other athletes ("other athletes," said as if I belong in the same category!) before heading to the bike transition area to meet Debbie off the bike, take ownership of our team's race chip and set off on the half marathon. I was expecting to be heading off around 12 noon, so I had all morning to relax and enjoy the event.

As Debbie would be relying on me to complete the race, I had been very careful with my kit the night before, not wanting to have any mishaps on race day. I wanted a good flat-lay photo, of course, but mostly I didn't want to let Debbie down. My bib number was carefully pinned onto my Massey club vest and then re-pinned four or five times until it was entirely straight and symmetrical. Having a running vest divided into quarters is somewhat triggering when you are a runner with slightly obsessive tendencies for neatness!

Even my socks were un-balled and laid flat on the bed because – life hack – it saves valuable seconds on race day not having to un-ball your socks!

Everything was ready to go and, after posting my flat-lay to Instagram, I climbed into bed, confident and with no pre-race anxieties. Other than that I was going to have to run a half marathon in the midday heat of central France, which was gripped by the worst heatwave in years – but that's a different story! I may write about it in a later chapter. (I say "may" because I might forget. It's really hard writing a book!)

After a couple of minutes in bed, I suddenly panicked that I didn't want to crease my bib number and risk looking scruffy in the official race photos, so I hopped back out of bed and carefully hung up my vest in the hotel wardrobe. I'm not sure how exactly it would have gotten creased laid out flat on the chair but such are the pre-race fears of a real runner who is just nodding off to sleep.

The next morning, I carefully packed all my kit into my bag and headed up to the race village, about 1.5 miles from my hotel. Ironman races, even half distances, start in the early hours of the morning so there is enough time for athletes to complete the mammoth overall distance. It is not uncommon for an athlete taking part in the full distance to be out for 14-16 hours, or 6-8 for those undertaking the half distance. After waving Debbie off into the water for her swim, I went out onto the course and had a great morning, cheering on athletes and catching glimpses of Debbie as she swam up and down the Allier River and then again as she made her way around the bike course.

Around 11am, I decided it was time to get ready. It would take me no more than 15 minutes to slip out of my clothes and into my race kit and I had an hour to spare (and, in all reality, longer because our timings were best case scenarios) but I really did not want to be late. One of my biggest fears was not being in transition when Debbie arrived after the bike leg and losing precious minutes of run time. Ironman events run to time. If you miss a cut-off, you are out!

At this particular event there were no changing rooms and I had to make do with changing in a portaloo. Unfortunately, my makeshift changing room had been in service since 5am that morning to the bowels of hundreds of nervous triathletes; bowels that had recently been under assault from last-minute attempts at carb-loading. (I could write a whole chapter on this one portaloo experience, and again I may well do, we'll have to see. I might leave something for a second book!)

It was cramped, and as I opened my bag, while holding my breath and trying not to let any part of me or anything I own touch the sides, floor or ceiling of the portaloo, I knew instantly something was wrong. I had a very immediate, intuitive sense that something was missing from my bag. I knew it was my vest before I even knew it was my vest – if that makes sense.

I did a bit of a comedy scramble through the bag just in case it was hidden. Maybe there was a mysterious pocket I had never noticed before and my vest was safely tucked away inside it? I was having a 'clutching at straws' moment! Like, "Could it be under that energy gel?" and "OMG, did I already unpack it and drop it into the toilet bowl?"

All my other bits and bobs were spilling out onto

the portaloo floor, which was muddy (hopefully it was mud), wet (hopefully it was not wee) and covered in flakes of tissue paper (hopefully all unused). I finished my frantic search with a final flourishing shake of the bag – just in case it was stuck in the bottom. In case you are wondering, the bag was not a cavernous Mary Poppins TARDIS of a bag. It was the size of a standard swimming bag that school children use. No way was a running vest going to be lurking in there, unseen to the naked eye.

But, as I said, I was clutching at straws.

After a few silent moments, it finally dawned on me, the very simple reason that my vest was not in the bag. I had left it hanging up in the hotel wardrobe. As I was frantically spilling my race kit over a dirty portaloo floor, my vest was hanging neatly in the wardrobe, crease-free, at the hotel a mile and a half away.

You can imagine my level of panic! I'm 2414 metres away from my vest and race bib (it sounds further in metres!), which I will not be permitted to race without, and there are approximately 45 minutes left until Debbie is expected back off the bike. I was more than a little frantic; I was sweating and very aware that there was absolutely no leeway in my run time that would allow me to go back and retrieve my vest and get back here in time to start and finish the half-marathon. As I mentioned, Ironman races are strictly timed and the finish line is closed the second the clock strikes the designated cut-off time. There's no medal for you if you're a few minutes late.

There was no chance of running without a bib number. The rules are not made to be broken in Ironman races. I burst forth from the portaloo, tears in my eyes (mostly from the vest issue; possibly some of it was due to portaloo fumes) and into the arms of a confused Stuart, who I hoped would have a bright idea to save the day!

Stuart and I had travelled to the race village that morning on our bikes to avoid parking charges, so a quick drive back to the hotel was out of the question. There was no way I could walk, run or cycle back to the hotel in time and getting out of the large park to find a taxi would have taken too long. Luckily, Stuart is a fast and competent cyclist who did not want to listen to me complain about one stupid kit mishap the rest of our lives. He hopped on his bike and pedalled for his life back over the bridge and towards our hotel. As he rode out of sight, I paced the park with nothing left to do but hope for the best. The next 30 minutes were very tense. If Debbie arrived now, we'd simply have to stand around making small talk and saying prayers that Stuart would make it back soon enough for me to run a half marathon in the ever-dwindling allotted time.

Luckily, he did – with maybe five minutes to spare – and when Debbie arrived, I was ready to greet her, in my crease-free vest, as if I'd been there waiting and well-prepared all along! She was none the wiser, although I have since confessed. I set off to run feeling relieved but possibly the least-prepared I have ever felt for any race ever.

Every time I mentioned to a running friend that I was writing a chapter that discussed running kit and clothes, I was met with a chorus of "Oooh, have you spoken to Daniel?"

Yes, I have spoken to Daniel!

It seems he has quite a reputation.

Daniel is a good friend of mine from my running club. He's a triathlete, an ultra-runner, a run coach as well as lots of other things, but he holds strong in one title over all others: The King of Kit Mishaps. I think at one point someone was going to make him a crown to wear. I even tried to get a new category invested into our running club awards; however, some of the committee felt it would be a landslide and not a particularly inclusive category, given Daniel's track record for kit mishaps.

There's one kit mishap involving a buff that I'm going to save for the toilet habits chapter later on as it's far more fitting for that topic. Actually, having said that, I think it's quite clear what this mishap involved just by mentioning 'buff' and 'toilet', so I don't think there's any more to add.

During the 'research' stage of this book (research is in inverted commas as it was mostly just me gossiping and chatting with running friends), I sat down with Daniel at our clubhouse after a training session and asked him how many races he'd managed to get through fully kitted out and without issue.

"I am not convinced I've had that many 'kit' disasters..." he told me, unwaveringly.

I noticed that he raised one eyebrow and I could see the cogs begin to turn in his mind as he started to recall examples of why he perhaps shouldn't be so keen to dismiss his newly-assigned title of King of Kit Mishaps.

He conceded that maybe he'd had one or two.

A little later that evening, my phone began to ping relentlessly with Facebook notifications. They were all from Daniel.

"Well, there was that time I left my running trainers at home so I ran parkrun in driving shoes. They were brogues, if I remember correctly."

Daniel is clearly not the kind of runner who will let a kit mishap stop him from running!

"I had forgotten my shorts and had to purchase a pair on the way to a marathon. Exactly the kind of new kit that should not be worn on race day, least of all marathon race day!"

Also not one to let a new piece of kit prevent the race from going ahead!

"Oh, how about the time I wore two different running shoes, as in a left shoe from one pair and a right shoe from another? Actually, that happened on more than one occasion. One time I styled it out as a fashion choice."

"Oooh and there was the time my running boxers split 1km into a race. I am notoriously too tight to bin them after only 1km of wear so I continued to run a further 41 kilometres in them. My inner thigh rubbed so badly it took a month to heal and required multiple visits to the nurse."

"Oooooooh I once ran a marathon in a running top that was still sweaty from parkrun that morning. It resulted in shredded nipples at 13 miles that bled so badly the blood showed through my purple top! An aid station volunteer was unable to treat me as it looked so bad. I have since been referred to as Nipples Man at a later incarnation of that event."

"Oooh oooh, there was the loss of a buff once – but that was far from a kit issue."

As mentioned.

"Ohhhhhh the time I did a marathon in plimsolls as I forgot my running shoes – actually, that wasn't too bad."

"Oh my gosh, I once ran a 4km in a sprint triathlon barefoot as the shoes were causing my foot serious pain. I had to carry the shoes on the run because leaving them in transition would have resulted in disqualification. That evening, upon further inspection of the shoes, I realised I had one of my son's Lego bricks under the inner sole."

"Oh yeah, I ran a race in a pair of black Speedos once as I picked up the wrong item of kit out of the drawer."

"Oh, that reminds me, I once ran in a Dracula outfit, complete with white face paint. It was a fantastic outfit to start with and I was lovely and warm on a cold day, with my PVC cape. I was only 1 mile in when I realised that wearing the least breathable, least sweat-wicking-away outfit ever created in the history of clothing design was not really that great an idea."

"Or that time at Junior parkrun, in my inflatable dinosaur costume, in the baking heat... It became so sweaty inside that I couldn't see where to run and was rescued seconds before I went into the River Avon. My hands got so swollen I couldn't undo the zip to get out! The fan that inflates and provides airflow was a lie! I also got stuck in the elasticated legs of the costume – which worked really well to keep the sweat inside and I found that it had pooled from the ankle to just below the knee."

To be fair, Daniel has done an awful lot of races so perhaps, relatively speaking, he's not had that many kit mishaps – but when you list them in the chapter of a book with no real context about his running career, it really does seem like he is a magnet for this kind of thing. Hopefully the list above provides a stark warning to others about the things that can and do go wrong with race day kit.

It seemed prudent in a chapter on kit to share with you some form of checklist that might help you avoid kit-related issues. Over time, Daniel has taken to producing his own kit checklist to help other runners not be so forgetful and it has been widely circulated around our running club (we're not sure he's using it himself yet though!), so I have added a snippet of it below, using both mine and Daniel's suggestions; a combined effort from two kit mishap survivors that hopefully prevents anyone else from having to borrow a stranger's spare trainers on race day (true story!).

Daniel and Jenna's Running Kit Checklist

✓ Running shoes – make sure these are well worn in and you are confident they provide the right level of support and comfort. Don't make the mistake of wearing brand new shoes for a race (do as Daniel says, not as he does!). It's always handy to have a spare set of laces with you too.

✓ Running top and bottoms – don't wear new gear, especially an item that could chafe on race day. You don't want to discover that it rubs in places you don't want it to rub, just when you don't need it to. Not only will you regret it during the race but you'll also regret it stepping into the shower later.

✓ Sports bra – if needed. Where possible, opt for a front-fastening one in case you need to get in or out of it in under two hours.

✓ A towel – for use if there are shower facilities at the end of the race or even just to towel yourself down when you're dripping with sweat. I, Jenna, personally also like a supply of baby wipes. Getting the crusty salt off my face at the end of a long hot race makes me feel human again, and less like a margarita.

- ✓ Bin bag or old jumper – it's good to keep warm on race day in between depositing your belongings and the klaxon sounding. Wear an old jumper or a bin bag to stay warm. Take care not to suffocate.
- ✓ Sunscreen and shades – you may well have been training in the cold and dark but remember, race day could end up being hot and sunny. In the UK, there's no telling what the weather will be like on race day. In Vichy when I, Jenna, set out to do the half marathon leg of the race, it was 41 degrees Celsius; however, a few years later when Penny (my amazing friend and inspiration for this book) was a spectator at the same event, it was 6 degrees at the same time of year and she had to purchase extra warm-weather clothes to make it through the trip!
- ✓ Vaseline – This can prove useful as a preventative for the nasty chafing that could occur, even in well-worn clothes (Daniel has added "particularly on the nipples" to this checklist item. I just want it to be 100% clear that this is a note from Daniel, not me!) or for post-race soothing.
- ✓ Muscle support, strapping, bandages and plasters – a small first aid kit with other essentials is useful should you have a mishap prior to the race or have a pre-existing issue that you need help with.
- ✓ Snack foods – bananas, cereal bars, chocolate and energy gels could all be useful additions but it is important not to eat anything on race day that you aren't used to, or you could spend more time with

the runs as opposed to actually running.

✓ Safety pins or magnets for your race number – you can never have too many of these and a lot of races don't provide them or if they do, they run out. Take enough for your friends just in case they forget theirs and you'll be a race day hero!

✓ Race number and race information – please read all the information provided by the organisers to make sure you aren't in the dark about anything. Secure your running number onto your top the night before. Just maybe leave it somewhere in plain sight, not hanging up in a closed wardrobe.

✓ Mobile phone – so you can meet up with your friends for a well-deserved drink at the end of the race or so they can let you know where they've found a spot to watch from. Or to call a taxi when your legs are too knackered to drive home after the race.

✓ Emergency cash – make sure you have some money to cover you in case of unforeseen circumstances or, if everything goes to plan, for a post-race ice-cream.

✓ Flip-flops – changing into a pair of flip-flops, or other breezy, comfortable shoes post-race, feels amazing on your feet! I, Jenna, made sure I had someone willing to peel off my socks after my marathon and help me into my flip-flops.

✓ Running watch – oops, nearly forgot that one!

If you've remembered to put on clothes for your race,

that's great, but the next problem to overcome is whether you are wearing the right clothes. Last night, a cold evening but a particularly sweaty training run, we all moaned about being too hot and one of the group shared some great advice from her own running experience: if you start a run warm, it's already too late for you!

It's obvious really when you think about it. She said that even though we are all quite scared to be cold at the start of a race and pile on the base layers, she has found that if she grins and bears the goose bumps and skin that is slowly turning blue, by the end of mile 1 she's perfectly comfortable. It's the same advice I got (and ignored) early on from one of the many Daves in my running club – dress for your second mile! I think it was you, Dave Goodwin, so thank you! (Dave, AKA 'The Boss', is our running club's trusty chairman!)

I'd like to build on this by saying that if you start a race not only warm, but super extra toasty warm, you are for sure going to have to do a mid-race strip. Just like I did one freezing November Sunday morning a few years ago. It was a flat and fast course and I was intending to go for a PB. However, it was so freezing cold that I felt I had to wear long thermal leggings, two base layers (yes, two) under my club vest, and my hat, gloves and buff. At the start, I was toasty. At mile 1, I was sweating through the base layers. At mile 3, you could have collected the sweat in buckets. It was mile 4 when I knew I had to lose some layers. The gloves and hat were thrown to a spectator (I got them back at the end; kit isn't cheap) and my buff went from around my neck to around my wrist. I wanted to finish the run in my club vest but I had to lose the layers underneath so, whilst keeping my pace up for the PB effort, I started peeling off the two base layers. Without taking off my vest? Whilst keeping up my PB attempt? Impossible!

Well, as it turned out, not impossible, just extremely difficult.

I eventually wrangled out of the two base layers, narrowly avoiding falling flat on my face, and I did get the PB I wanted. It was just unfortunate that the race photographer caught a shot of me mid-strip, my head and left arm stuck in a base layer, flashing the right side of my sports bra and belly flab to the camera. I haven't told you which race it was, and I won't, but just know the photo is still out there. There is also a photo of me vomiting up an orange at the finish line. My other mistake of the day was to think that citrus fruit would make a good pre-race, PB attempt breakfast. Huge thanks to Cathy and James, who comforted me in my time of need. Shame on Stuart and the other Cathy, who laughed at me as I publicly vomited up a juicy orange!

I made that whole de-robing very difficult for myself in order to preserve my PB attempt (I could have just stopped running and taken the layers off) but there is something far trickier to manoeuvre into and out of – and that is the dreaded sports bra. Those runners who are in need of a sports bra will know how real the struggle is, although there is some debate about which is harder – putting on a sports bra (and getting it in the right position so you can run comfortably) or taking off a sweaty sports bra, post-run.

I personally think the former is worse – I usually spend five minutes holding it up in front of my puzzled face, trying to work out where the straps should go before temporarily dislocating my wrists to get it done up at the back. (I have only recently discovered front-fastening sports bras. My life has changed!)

As my fabulous running friend Jane points out though, you're not sweating too much at this point. She believes it's far worse to have to remove the entangled web of straps post-run when you are hot, sweating and knackered. She may be right. I've heard that for many runners, the post-run removal of a sports bra has become a two-man job!

When my lovely friend Julie overheard me talking about my flashing incident above, she said: "Well, here's a story you'll definitely want to include in your book," and she was not wrong!

Julie told me of the time her father, an excellent, accomplished runner, was leading a race and rounded the corner towards the finish line to an abundance of cheers from the crowd, which included Julie and her brother. At first glance, Julie was thrilled to see her dad winning. At second glance, she noticed he was… let's say 'exposed' in the shorts area. Not wanting him to risk violating public decency laws (or end up with some very dodgy finish line photos), over the crowds Julie shouted, as loud as she could, "Dad, your willy is out!"

Julie's dad, being a consummate professional, took a quick glance downwards and, without losing any speed, discretely tucked everything away and went on to win the race in a dignified manner.

Well done, that man!

It got me thinking though about how 'aware' I am at the end of the race – particularly should I be winning, not that it would ever happen. If Julie was at the finish line, waving at me and shouting: "Jenna, your fanny is out!" would I even hear her or register the words? I'm fairly oblivious to what is going on around me when I'm running flat-out and nearing the finish line. I'd probably just wave back, assuming they were supportive clubmate cheers; I might even throw my arms in the air or maybe perform a little jump (which would make it entirely worse!). I'd probably cross the line with some kind of over-the-top finish line pose, grinning and basking in the perceived glory, entirely oblivious to my indecent exposure, which is certainly being caught on camera.

My brain has gone straight to the fashion show scene in *The Inbetweeners*…

Thinking about accidental exposure in running got me wondering about organised nudity in running. I vaguely know that naked running exists. I am by no means an expert.

I started my 'research' in the simplest way by Googling 'naked running'. I found myself faced with a host of YouTube videos, memes, images and sign-up websites to get involved in various naked runs across the world. I naively assumed a naked run would be on the more conservative and less literal side and would be running in maybe just pants, or at least running with strategically-placed cover-ups, but no, there are many runs around the world in which you take part fully nude.

Nothing to hide!

It begs a few questions:

Q: Is there an optimum place to keep one's timing chip?

Q: Where does one pin one's race number?

Q: Is the lack of sports bra an issue for those who normally need one?

Q: Would any gender have more of an advantage, anatomically and aero-dynamically speaking?

Q: Are there naked relay races? What are the risks of running naked with a baton?

Q: Is it easier to pack for a race where you need no clothes?

Q: Do runners travel to the start line naked or strip off on the line?

Q: Are the volunteers naked?

Q: Do naked races only take place in the summer? Who wants to run naked in the cold, but then again who wants to get sunburnt somewhere sensitive?

Q: Would you rather be at the front of the pack with everyone looking at your bum or the back of the pack looking at everyone else's bums?

Q: Do normal words of encouragement between runners get exchanged as 'compliments' i.e. instead of "Well done, keep going," do you hear "Nice bum, keep going!"?

Q: Do you get a race T-shirt? Do participants realise the irony of that?

Q: Is there a race photographer? Have they been vetted?

If you think I'm going to answer all these questions here in this book, I'm sorry to disappoint you. I think the only way to know must be to take part and the only naked run I have ever done is the midnight dash from the bedroom to the bathroom! I'll leave you to do your own research. You might want to try Google (although not on your work computer like I did!) or maybe even sign up for a naked race yourself. If you do, please let me know how you get on. Apparently, it doesn't feel seedy or like you might be subject to objectification; apparently, it just feels very normal once you are there – I can't tell you who told me this but I have it on good authority!

I was looking for a neat way to finish this section on running kit before moving onto the next chapter regarding toilet habits and, serendipitously, my fabulous running friend Joy just provided me with the following funny anecdote involving both kit and weeing (yes, it's about a dog weeing and not a runner, but it counts!).

During an outdoor RaceFit session, Joy found herself feeling a little overheated, so she pulled off her expensive branded club hoody and placed it carefully over a bollard in the park. It's worth noting that our local park is rife with dog walkers at this time of the evening, and they do wander fairly close to the RaceFit location (the car park!) to have a nosy at what is going on. 20+ runners dressed in hi-vis and lunging around a car park does attract attention…

Joy was mid-squat (this is very likely to be untrue; I just like the notion that Joy was possibly mid-squat when she noticed the following occur) and glanced over towards where her hoody was situated to see, quite unexpectedly, a dog cocking his leg up the bollard and peeing all over her hoody. What's more, the dog's owner was watching her beloved doggo's actions like it was totally OK and acceptable! Joy actually had to point out to the walker that her dog was relieving himself over her expensive piece of kit and ask her if she would mind incredibly if that could be stopped…

Race Report
Nicola's Polar Night Half Marathon

Tromsø, Norway

This time last week, 5th January 2019, I was 217 miles north of the Arctic Circle in Tromsø, Norway (69 degrees north), having travelled about 1,400 miles north just to run a half marathon.

Fast forward to today, 12th January, and I'm at home on the sofa in Coventry (52 degrees north), wrapped in blankets, with a heavy cold and chesty cough, wondering if last weekend really happened.

I've been a bit obsessed with the Polar Night Half, and its sister race the Midnight Sun Marathon, for a while. I love Norway, visit frequently, and as I got back into running over the last three years a plan began to evolve that I might actually be able to enter these races. I decided that if I could complete a couple of half marathons in 2018 I'd go ahead and enter the Polar Night Half. With both Stratford and Kenilworth half marathons complete, I felt confident to enter the race, but I didn't really know what I was letting myself in for. A quick bit of research showed I would need to be prepared to run in temperatures which would most likely be around -5°C (with a 'feels like' temperature most likely in negative double figures), that it was likely to snow, and I'd probably need spikes. Not to mention a lot of layers. It was starting to feel like a bit of an expedition.

I started training in the autumn, and also started to

get the kit together. I soon realised that whilst I could easily layer up on my top half, I was going to need better leggings and socks to stay warm (or should that be to not completely freeze). Windproof thermal compression leggings and knee-length stay-dry (ha!) thermal socks were sourced. I'd read that there is always debate on the start line of the race: spikes or no spikes. As I don't own any spikes, I was glad to discover some spikes that were attached to a rubber sole that you could pull over your normal trainers. Problem solved. And when it came to the race, boy was I glad to have those on board!

Finally, the day came for me to set off to Norway. I'd been keeping an eye on the weather forecast and was a little disappointed to see that temperatures were predicted to be slightly above freezing! This wasn't the Arctic vision I'd imagined. However, I arrived in Tromsø to find ice! Norway obviously doesn't grind to a halt in these conditions, but nevertheless, I was terrified I'd fall and injure myself before even getting to the start line. Luckily, my worst fears didn't transpire.

Race day didn't dawn (the sun doesn't rise in Tromsø from mid-November to mid-January), and I went to pick up my race number. There were hundreds of people milling around, and I spoke with people from all over the world who had travelled for the race: Australians, Americans, Germans, Irish, Dutch… and eight people from Coventry, including two from Northbrook, another running club local to me! It was great to hear everyone's stories and the excitement was building. I treated myself at the merchandise stall to a long-sleeved T-shirt and a hat.

The race began at 3pm, so there was some time to get nervous! I had lunch and then went back to get changed for the start. I don't think I've ever worn so many clothes to run in: thermal base layer, T-shirt, windproof coat, Massey Running Club vest, hat, a couple of buffs, gloves, mittens, thermal leggings and thermal socks. As it was, the 'feels like' temperature for the race was about -3°C and rather windy in places. I'd say I got the kit on the cold side of correct – one more layer would have been too much, but there were times when I was very cold.

There was a mass warm-up in the square just before 3pm, and then we all piled into the start funnel. From there, there was no messing around: within a couple of minutes the countdown had begun and we were off! It was pitch dark, and Tromsø's main street was lined with people and lit with beautiful twinkly garlands with a red heart in the middle hanging across the street. There was excitement in the air, and I forgot to start my watch as I tried to take it all in. There was lots of support, and the Norwegians were all shouting, "Hej ja! Hej jah!" and ringing cowbells in encouragement. There were 2,400 places for the race, and I'd read that over 2,000 places were sold – however, only around 1,000 of us lined up on the starting line.

Immediately I was glad of the over-shoe spikes, as

the road was icy. The organisers had been advising everyone to wear spikes because of the conditions, and we sounded like a mass tap-dancing troupe click-clacking down the street. The course is an out-and-back course, beginning on Storgata (the main street) and heading out to the airport before heading back along the same route. After running through the main street, we ran along paths past some very pretty houses – typical Norwegian wooden clapboard properties with fairy lights in the windows and welcome lanterns by the doors. There were lots of people out supporting the runners so the atmosphere was great. From there, the route came out onto a closed road, and in places the route was lit by flaming torches. Parts of the route were right next to the fjord, which was frozen near the shore.

The halfway point was at the airport, where it was also windiest. At this point I was worried I'd got the kit all wrong as I was absolutely frozen. Conditions underfoot varied from ice, slush and snow to gritty tarmac and freezing icy puddles, which were too much even for Drymax socks, and I had cold, wet feet. There were drink stations every 5k, with energy drinks and lukewarm water. I never thought I'd enjoy lukewarm water during a race, but it was perfect!

Just after the turning point, I had a low mile with shooting pain down my right leg, so I had no choice but to switch to stretch, walk, run, repeat for a bit until it eased off enough to get back to running. By this time, the wind had got up and it was pretty cold, but

I was still ridiculously excited to be there and just focused on keeping going. Any thoughts of a target time had gone out of the window by now; the mission was to get it done. There were no distance markers on the course until the last 5km, so when I saw that 5km sign, I knew I was going to do it. Just a parkrun to go! I couldn't stop smiling, and I knew I couldn't stop running. I was literally grinning from ear to ear for the last 5km, and waving to the marshals and passing pedestrians, who must've thought I was mad.

I'll never forget the feeling of coming onto the main street with the finish arch in sight, grinning like mad, somehow finding a bit of a kick to give it the best finish I could manage, knowing that I was about to achieve something from my bucket list. To top it all, just before I crossed the line, I heard a roar of "Go Massey!" and realised it came from one of the Northbrook guys I'd met earlier in the day. That really meant a lot, up there in the Arctic on my own.

I was handed my medal (which looks like it has the Northern Lights inside it) and a volunteer wrapped me in a foil blanket. I got some hot juice and was directed into the Sami lavvu (traditional tent) to warm up around a fire pit. Definitely like no other race I've ever entered! I'm so looking forward to going back to run the Midnight Sun Marathon. All being well, this will be my first marathon.

The race was well marshalled and runners were prioritised over drivers at junctions, which was good to see. Norwegian drivers take this with good grace too. Sadly it was too cloudy to glimpse the Northern Lights, and to be honest, I was concentrating so hard on putting one foot in front of the other without falling over, I'm not sure I'd have noticed them if they had been visible! The spikes did give me confidence to run fairly freely once I'd got used to them though.

If you are thinking of doing this race, bear in mind that Norway is super-expensive. My race entry fee of around 600NOK (about £60) didn't include a T-shirt, only a medal. There is a 10k and a 5k race run at the same time, so if you're travelling with others who don't want to run a half, there's options for them too. All in all, I highly recommend this as an incredible experience.

Chapter Four
Toilet Habits

During the early stages of writing this book, I spoke to my magnificent and knowledgeable friend Wendy who advised that any book on what running really looks like needs at least a whole chapter on 'wild weeing'.

Of course, Wendy is absolutely right – so here it is!

Just quickly, before I go any further, please remember that public urination (or worse) has all sorts of legal, moral, ethical and ecological implications. Take what you read here with a pinch of salt and when you have to go mid-run, don't do anything that would upset, disrupt or disgust passers-by, land owners or Mother Nature. Or the police!

Amongst runners, wild weeing, if you haven't heard the phrase, refers to having a mid-run wee in an open public place somewhere along your run route. It may or may not require the use of natural materials in lieu of toilet paper, for example a large soft leaf or a handful of grass. (NB The need to use such materials may depend largely on your anatomy. Some runners may need nothing more than a quick shake.)

During our discussion, Wendy went on to explain that in her experience the backbone of a good wild wee is location! Location! Location! Her own top tip is:

"Find a spot that looks out onto a field of

bluebells."

By opting for a field of bluebells, or of course any wildflower meadow of your choosing, you'll benefit in a number of ways:

- You will have something nice to look at while you wee
- It will be cathartic, therapeutic and calming to feel surrounded by the presence of nature as you do what nature intended
- Passers-by will think you are simply admiring the view and will be oblivious to what you are actually doing

Note that point three above only really applies to those runners blessed with the ability to wee standing up. For those amongst us who need to squat or crouch, that would clearly be a very odd stance to take whilst admiring a field of bluebells and I don't think anyone would believe you were just flower-spotting in that particular position.

During the early stages of writing this chapter, I bumped into two of my very good running friends in the car park of the Excel gym in Coventry. (Don't worry, I don't work out. I'm not a gym bunny. I was there to get a Covid test!)

After lots of pleasantries and small talk, having not seen each other for over a year because of the lockdowns, they mentioned they had only stopped there to take a quick comfort break and use the facilities. I felt bad pointing out that the gym, including the loos, was closed because of the pandemic.

"Not to worry," my male friend said, casually. "I'll find a hedge."

Without a flinch, he moved from Plan A to Plan B (or should that be Plan Pee?). No sense of fear or panic because, as a male, the mid-run peeing process is very straightforward. And quick. For male runners, their shorts don't need to come fully down and they can get nice and close to their chosen hedge – their non-prickly, non-poisonous chosen hedge – when making their mid-run pit stop. And although passers-by might know exactly what they are doing, they probably won't get an eyeful of something private.

For us female runners, it's not so straightforward. The shorts almost always have to come fully down, revealing a pasty pair of cheeks in the process. At best, they might not be pasty. Then a squat or hunch of some sort is usually needed and that is what makes it difficult to disguise what you are doing.

I personally have never had a wild wee! You might be thinking that before writing about wild weeing, a legitimate author would do some field research on the subject (like going for a wee in a field?) but as I'm sure you're starting to figure out, this book was not written on copious amounts of research. It was written from experience and/or lack of experience in some cases. I'm quite happy writing about wild weeing while having no experience of it whatsoever.

Although, that being said, I have witnessed a lot of other runners' wild wees.

By chance, I should add. Not by voyeurism.

For example, at my local parkrun, there is a spot en route that delves off into the adjacent woods and over time there has developed a distinctly parkrunner-shaped hole in the foliage. The proximity of the run route to the hedge, and the reluctance of parkrunners to go too far into the woods and lose further valuable seconds, means that every Saturday I get to watch wild weeing in action. And that is more than enough research for me!

On a recent club training run, my fabulous cousin and fellow running club member Emma listened as I explained that I was looking for runners' experiences of wild weeing. She told me she knew of a great tip for when you want to have a mid-run wee, unnoticed.

I was all ears, not because I do much wild weeing (as I said, I've never indulged) but because I was keen to lock in a tip for my, at that time, hypothetical future readers. Also, Emma is something of a motivational expert – every day she shares a heartfelt and life-affirming quote or piece of advice to keep up the spirits of her friends and family. I knew she'd have something good to share!

"Go on then, Emma, let's hear it!" I said.

"You squat down," she started.

"Yeah," a few of us replied, intrigued to hear the next steps.

"You whip your knickers down."

"Yeah," we replied again, still intrigued.

"You take your phone out."

"Er, where are you going with this, Emma?" I whispered to her, not sure what to expect next and also mildly concerned about where she keeps her phone during a run.

"You hold your phone up in the air," Emma continued to explain.

"With both hands or just one?" I asked, curious.

"It's not important!" she told me.

"OK," came my reply.

NB There are not many opportunities for dialogue in a book like this, so I'm eking this out a bit, to be honest.

Emma began to summarise: "So, you're squatting, your pants are down, your phone is in the air. At this point you can start peeing and as you do, start taking some photos. People will simply think you are taking a photo from a clever, professional angle and the shutter noise will distract from the whoosh of your wee."

The running crew stood silent for a moment, taking on board Emma's suggestion.

Eventually, after some thinking time, our ever-conscientious running friend Heather pointed out that you really need to be confident you've got your camera facing the right way for this one or you'll end up with a somewhat voyeuristic photo album on your phone.

Another top tip: don't swipe right on Emma's phone, just in case!

I've since had some time to think about Emma's

suggestion and I think it's brilliant, but I have some concerns that I'd like to address at some point:

- What if passers-by notice the trail of urine?
- What if passers-by don't notice the trail of urine and wander over to you and it runs over their shoes?
- What if a passer-by stops to ask you a photography-related question?
- What if they genuinely think you are taking a photo and in turn take a photo of you for one of those arty photo-of-a-photo shots?

I may be something of an overthinker at times…

A few other top tips I came across when discussing this subject with my running friends:

- Wee downhill of your feet – unless you want to end up in a warm offensive puddle
- Check which way the wind is blowing (This might only be relevant to those opting for a stand-up wee. You should be out of the wind if you are going with the squat)
- Speed is your friend. Going fast means less time to be spotted and fewer splashes, and a fast stream flows straighter, meaning less chance of soggy shoes

Following on from Emma's lesson in covert wild weeing, the lovely Lianne admitted that all her past attempts at wild weeing have had to be aborted mid-stream. Each time she had worked up the courage to have a go, a passer-by had appeared out of nowhere. The threat of this is something that came up regularly amongst all the runners I spoke to who have been caught short mid-run.

Here's how the story generally goes, so I'm told.

You spend quite a bit of time sussing out the ideal spot. You can run for 1-2 miles before finally settling on a spot that suits your needs. Will it be a hedge, a tree, a bush? (Are you also childish enough to snigger at the word bush?) Once you have settled on a spot and resigned yourself to getting your bits out in the fresh air, you check, check, and check again that there is no one in sight to catch you. Once you are in position and just prior to lowering your shorts, you check, check, and check again to make sure there is still no one around to catch you. There isn't a person in sight for miles. And then…

As you are meagre seconds away from passing the point of no return, someone comes along, whistling and blissfully happy because their day hasn't yet been ruined by the sight of a stranger urinating in public. You have to abort your wild wee, abruptly and at speed, and spend more uncomfortable miles sussing out the next suitable location. Of course, by this point the only thing you can think about is having a wee, so your run is effectively ruined.

Not all running wees are 'wild' and at organised races, runners are usually blessed with facilities of some sort. If you're lucky you might be racing at a sports ground, track or 'real' venue that has the 'luxury' of a real toilet – I say luxury, it's probably still pretty basic.

I doubt there's a person in there gently offering you an Egyptian cotton towel for your hands and wafting a spritz of Chanel No. 5 as you leave, but it's an actual porcelain toilet with a seat, nonetheless.

If you're unlucky, you'll find yourself in a portaloo. When it comes to juggling a run with a call of nature, I'm sure that most of us would agree that portaloos are one of the least enjoyable elements we have to contend with.

The first portaloo problem is the queuing. All the quintessentially British queuing etiquette, the queuing rules widely held by society, go out of the window when it comes to standing in line for a portaloo at a race. The main confusion seems to be that half the runners in the queue are under the impression that there's one queue for **ALL** the portaloos whilst the remaining runners are lining up individually for **EACH** portaloo. Mass confusion and chaos ensues. Personally, I always end up doing a little dance I call The Portaloo Queue Shuffle!

Imagine you are in the main queue, patiently waiting for the next available portaloo. After what seems like an eternity, you finally reach the front and see a door swing open. You move towards the door but, from the corner of your eye, you see the runner at the front of the individual queue for that loo move forward and duck in before you. So you step back and cast your eyes down the line of loos. A door at the other end swings open. You make a move but the new runner now at the front of the main queue gets there first. It's like bloody portaloo hokey cokey. You are stuck in no-man's land with neither queue seeming to work for you. After a few minutes of doing this merry little dance, hopping back and forth between loos, you decide to change tack and join the back of one of the individual queues. As you reach the front and the door directly ahead of you swings open, someone from the main queue dashes in. Arrghhh!

Try to stay calm if this happens to you. Chances are you don't really need a wee – you just nervously think you do!

If you do eventually make it into a portaloo, the next problem to overcome is the decision to sit or hover. Let's do pros and cons.

Sitting pros
- Your legs won't ache as much
- You will have more control over directional flow
- You can enjoy a moment of quiet reflection
- Your running shoes will remain splash-free

Sitting cons
- You are just that bit closer to the contents of nervy race-day bowels from around the country. Bowels that, for the last week, have existed on a diet of pizza, baked potatoes, toast, energy drinks and coffee (because, you know, they've been carb-loading)

Hover pros
- No part of your skin will come into contact with the warm, germ-riddled toilet seat

<u>Hover cons</u>

- Your legs may start to shake
- You risk getting your running shoes wet... That is, if they are not already wet because you're in there following someone who peed all over the floor!
- It is less relaxing

If you still can't decide what to do after running through the pros and cons list, you'll often find that the vacating runner will share a word of wisdom, for example:

"It's not looking so good in there."

Or:

"You might want to give that one a miss."

But do you take their word for it?

You don't really have many options at this point. Plus, it's always possible that whilst loo number two isn't looking its best, loo number six could be so much worse...

Once you have secured a portaloo, made your choice between sitting and hovering and finally finished doing what you needed to do, your last hurdle is to decide whether to enlist the pointless 'flush'.

Flushing is polite; however, in a portaloo it is like pulling the lever on a very disgusting Vegas slot-machine. There are no winners. Even after you have vigorously wiggled the lever back and forth five times there is still no jackpot. It has done nothing to disperse the contents of the bowl.

All that you have left to do now is step back outside into the real world and pray that someone from the portaloo company has just installed a row of sparkling white porcelain sinks, with toasty hot water and Jo Malone English Pear and Freesia handwash. Maybe there's even a matching hand moisturiser!

But just so you know, they never have and there never is.

All you will find outside the portaloo is a bank of makeshift plastic sinks and agitated runners aggressively pumping the foot pedal, desperately trying to get a single droplet of freezing cold water that will in no way make them feel clean again, let alone destroy any bacteria they picked up in the portaloo. Basically, the whole portaloo experience will likely result in you contracting gastroenteritis and in less than 12 hours, you'll be vomiting into an old basin next to your bed.

All for a wee you probably didn't even need!

At least you'll be able to console yourself with a race goody bag full of irrelevant leaflets and 5% off money vouchers for products you'll never buy.

One runner, who would like to remain nameless – and you'll see why – revealed to me their own portaloo horror story. It was at a half marathon race but they have forgotten which one. Personally, I think they just fear there is more chance of identification if they reveal too many of the finer details.

After concluding their business in the portaloo, they inexplicably (their word) stood up and turned around, perhaps with morbid curiosity, and inspected the contents of the bowl. They bent down further to get a better look.

"Why?" I interrupted when they got to this part of their story, and they honestly had no idea why.

In a blur, mid-bend, they felt a gust of wind whistle through a gap in the slightly warped door frame of the portaloo. (So it's at a windy venue... hmmm... Silverstone Half Marathon?) A door which they had only slightly locked due to portaloo claustrophobia. Overcome by the gust of wind, the lock slid out of its safe haven and the door blew wide open, revealing the runner, bare-bottomed, peering into the depths of portaloo hell. In front of an orderly queue of runners waiting their turn.

Apparently, no one said anything.

Interestingly, this person ran a PB that day, presumably in a bid to get the whole thing over and done with, get home and never see anyone from that race again. Ever.

During a race a few years back, I set off and within the first mile I genuinely needed a wee – not a pretend pre-race fake wee, but a real wee. Thinking back, I'm not sure how it happened as I had tinkled four or five times in the pre-race wee section of the day.

I rounded a corner on a dull lifeless industrial estate (it was a beautiful race in parts, just not all the parts) and spotted a single portaloo with a small queue. To this day, I'm not entirely sure it was a race-sanctioned portaloo as it seemed out of place, in an entirely random and bizarre spot. I do still worry that it was some form of weirdo exhibitionist facility and everyone who used it was live-streamed across the internet for the viewing pleasure of the world's perverts.

If any of the perverts reading this come across it on the web, please let me know.

The genuineness of the portaloo aside, my dilemma mid-race was that this was supposed to be a 10k PB attempt for me. I had two choices: stop, wee and risk losing my PB, or hold it in, keep aiming for the PB but spend the next 45 minutes in increasing discomfort.

The trouble I have is that once I have allowed a single lone 'wee' thought to creep in, my internal voice begins a monotonous chant of "Wee! Wee! Wee! Wee!" in time to the patter of my feet on the ground. I was running pretty fast (for me), so it was quite a distracting chant. There was no tuning it out, so I opted for a loo break, despite my PB attempt, and joined the queue.

Despite doing everything right in said queue…
- I hopped from foot to foot
- I looked around anxiously
- I checked my watch continuously
- I repeatedly said: "Come on, come on!" so everyone knew I was in a rush

…I did not get a PB that day.

I suppose I did enjoy the race, so that's the main

thing, but I say that begrudgingly because I still really wanted the PB!

A more recent trend that has sprung up in the toilet industry (is it a whole industry?) are female urinals. I have experienced these for myself, at the London Marathon. At the expo I was supplied with my goodie bag, which contained a 'handy' flatpack urinary device (just what everyone expects to receive in their race goodie bag!) and I was instructed that when the time comes (to wee) I should just unfold the device, build the sides according to the instructions and hey presto! I would find myself with my very own peeing funnel.

If you've not used one before, the best way I can describe it is as follows.

Have you ever ordered a single slice of pizza – I bet you are wondering where I am going with this – maybe in America or from a street vendor, and that slice of pizza has been served on a flat piece of carboard wider at one end, tapering down into a point (so pretty much pizza-shaped!) and with small sides to hold your pizza in place?

A pee funnel is basically one of those. A pizza holder.

I wonder if the company that manufactures pee funnels and the company that manufactures pizza holders have ever identified the cross-over in markets?

To use a pee funnel is quite straightforward, in

theory. You simply position the wider end beneath your crotch, direct the pointy end towards the urinal and you're good to go. For me though, it was easier said than done and I really struggled to use it. Not physically – there's nothing wrong with me – but I had a real mental block as well as a crisis of confidence. I absolutely did not want to pull my running shorts down in front of all these other runners. And I definitely did not want them to see, hear or even know I was peeing. Although what else would I have been doing there in the female urinals? Of course, I realise the other runners were not looking at me, had no interest in me and hopefully were all there for the same reason as me: one of many pre-marathon nervous wees.

Nonetheless, I spent over 20 minutes standing in close proximity to the urinals considering my options. Well, I say options plural but I didn't really have a whole host of them. It was either go now or succumb to plan B: hold it in for the next six hours.

With a marathon ahead of me, I really had no choice and when I finally plucked up the courage to go, I can honestly say it was the worst wee of my life. I felt exposed, awkward, weird. I realise now that all of my wees since I was a child have been in private, so of course this al fresco group setting was going to be difficult. It didn't feel particularly sanitary either. As always, the hand-washing station consisted of freezing cold water and a tiny soap dispenser that had run out after the tenth dispense, never to be refilled again.

One of the things that I was most unimpressed with, though, was the privacy (or should that be lack of privacy?) of the female urinals. The 'walls' of the urinal zone consisted of 6ft railings to which PVC-type material had been zip-tied around the outside. This meant there were gaps. Big gaps. All the way around!

The edges of the material didn't quite meet. Bits were flapping open (apologies if that feels like a questionable choice of words in a paragraph about female urinals) and I'm quite confident that any dirty running peeper could get a good eyeful, should they want to. And let's face it, there are 40,000 runners in the area that day. One of them is bound to be a bit dodgy!

The London Marathon is the only race where I have been for one, and only one, pre-race wee...

A lot of what we've discussed so far has been number one oriented. Naturally, we have a second matter to discuss. Matter number two.

Last year, I was spectating and supporting at a triathlon race and had placed myself somewhere along the multi-lap run route to cheer everyone on. Early on in the race, I spotted one of the front-ish runners with a fairly panicked look on their face. By front-ish, I mean they were not going to win the race but they were certainly a clear 20 miles ahead of where I would be at that point.

While other runners were head down, plugging

away, this panic-stricken runner swerved off the route and began zig-zagging across the field, his eyes darting from side to side as he repeatedly uttered one single word, his voice tinged with panic as he pleaded with spectators to help him find what he was looking for:

"Toilet?"

"Toilet?"

"Toilet!"

With each gasp, he sounded more and more desperate. It eventually became less of a question and more of a demand:

"TOILET!!!!"

He was sweating quite profusely and I could see tears pricking his eyes.

All at once, in perfect harmony, I and the other spectators gave him the answer he so desperately wanted.

"Over there!" we chorused, simultaneously pointing towards the bank of portaloos just over yonder.

As he darted off towards the portaloos, completely unable to thank us, I noticed that his run had become more of an awkward limp. As the spectators all turned back to watch the race, I heard one quiet but wise voice whisper:

"When you gotta go, you gotta go."

Followed by one even wiser spectator who said:

"I think he already went."

I never saw the runner again. In fact, thinking

about it, I don't recall seeing him come out of the portaloo. Perhaps he was too embarrassed.

During a conversation with a group of runners – half very proper, half absolutely feral – about the worst things they have done in a bid to relieve themselves mid-run, I noticed that some of the very proper runners would baulk at the shenanigans of the others and state, with some disgust, "Well, I've never done such a thing!" and it prompted me to include *Never Have I Ever: The Runner's Edition* in this book.

I don't know if you've heard of this game, so I'll briefly explain how it usually works. You get a group of slightly drunk adults together and sit them in a circle. The first person begins by saying: "Never have I ever…" and then states something they've never done whilst running. Those in the group who have done it take a shot of something alcoholic and, in doing so, reveal their distasteful behaviour to the others. After a few seconds of shock, mocking, giggling and red faces, the second person takes their go and begins "Never have I ever…" and so on until everyone gets bored, runs out of things to say or falls asleep drunk.

Never have I ever played this game (see what I did there?) but here are my suggested never-have-I-evers to get the game started:

- Never have I ever used my running buff as toilet paper.
- Never have I ever used my running gloves as

toilet paper.
- Never have I ever used leaves as toilet paper.
- Never have I ever used a stranger's toilet on route.
- Never have I ever popped into a pub to use the toilet.
- Never have I ever used a portaloo during a run.
- Never have I ever been caught wild weeing.
- Never have I ever shit myself on a run.

And so on…

We know runners like to drink, so introducing a drinking game is open to abuse. I know of at least 50 runners who would be downing shots after every round regardless of whether they'd done said deed or not! However, that is part of the fun. Just make sure you always play this game post-run. Never before!

And doing things that no one else ever has brings me nicely on to a race report from my brilliant friend Janette. A race report that is most definitely, very specifically related to the content of this chapter. If Janette ever plays Never Have I Ever and uses the scenario from her race report, I suspect she will win hands down!

Race Report
Janette's Cotswolds Hilly 100

It will be fun, they said!

A real race after a long pandemic of solo running and virtual races.

All you have to do is show up in a country lane miles from home where you meet a runner at about 7.30am, grab a baton from them and literally run for the hills, try not to get lost and pass your baton on some 10 miles later.

OK, well I like a little hill, I thought to myself (and, perversely prefer to run up them than down them).

"I'm in!" I said.

During the driving recce of the route, I felt a sinking feeling when I realised there were not going to be any portaloos anywhere, just a public toilet midway through my route which might not even be open before 9am on a sleepy Sunday morning.

But no worries, hey ho, there's always a bush to be found, right?

Well yes, if you can pole-vault over one into a field, and don't mind the hawthorns or the barbed wire. And pardon me for being precious but I'm not risking a rip to my favourite dayglo orange shorts under any circumstances.

So, tossing and turning the night before the big day, having purchased a 'she-wee' to take care of Problem Number One (ladies, trust me, these are ace), my thoughts turned to the elephant in the room that is

Problem Number Two.

What would Bear Grylls do? I thought.

Well, he would take a little trowel and dig a little hole, etcetera, but perhaps not on a pretty grass verge or near a meeting point rammed with runners' cars and, well, runners!

Lots of runners. Everywhere.

All over the place.

OK. So I get up at six, eat my Shreddies, put my running kit on, dispense with Problem Number One (the easy peasy problem) whilst still at home, grab my Thermos-packed coffee fix and head for the race, hoping for the best. By 6:20am I am in the car, with a heightened sense of anxiety knowing that the race is now underway and some poor soul is on their way to our meeting point to hand me the baton while I still haven't figured out Problem Number Two.

But I am resourceful, and I've told myself to think outside the box. And then I have a lightbulb moment:

"A BOX!"

So there I find myself, at 7:10am, amid the melee of runners, wedged between my car and a hedge, with a large blanket wrapped around me.

"Poor chick, she looks like she's cold," is what I hope other runners were thinking.

But what I am actually doing is squatting, remarkably comfortably, over a shallow plastic storage box, which is lined with a pedal-bin liner (obviously), and I'm saying a prayer!

I'm actually feeling like Harry Potter under his

invisibility cloak.

One minute or so later and let's say Problem Number Two is no more.

I'm a tidy person, I like my ducks in a row and the countryside is left as beautiful as I found it that morning.

So there you have it. I took my baton at 7:26am and bounded off feeling light as a feather, running for the hills.

Chapter Five
Always Read the Race Pack

As a new runner, I certainly learned the hard way about many aspects of the sport. Like why running uphill very fast in cheap trainers is bad for your Achilles tendon.

I found that my new running friends, who were all far more experienced than I was, very kindly just wanted to encourage me and help me to advance. I was met with lots of "Just go for it!" and "You can do it!" when I wanted to do stupid things like run a marathon just because I'd recently watched the movie *Run Fatboy Run*.

It seemed like nobody wanted to tell me the bad things to look out for – which I do find odd, as runners usually jump at the chance to impart knowledge or discuss their past injuries, mishaps and faux pas.

When it comes to rookie mistakes, my favourite is a story entitled *Stuart's First Marathon*.

I should mention this is my aforementioned other half Stuart, not any of my other running friends named Stuart, before any of them start panicking!

In 2009, Stuart entered the ballot for the 2010 London Marathon. This was back in the day when the ballot opened at midnight and automatically closed after a certain number of ballot entries were processed. You had to watch the clock tick over painfully slowly, sick with nervous butterflies and the fear that your internet would suddenly go down at 11:59 and you'd miss out on a ballot place.

A ballot place.

That is all you were vying for – not an entry in the race, just a position on a teetering cliff edge of mixed emotion for the next five months until they announced the lucky few who had successfully nabbed an actual real place.

Stuart only entered the ballot because his mum Julie – she'll enjoy a name drop – really wanted to do the London Marathon as a bucket-list challenge after years of watching it on the television.

Stuart, being the kind, devoted, loving son that he is, thought he'd support his mum and enter the ballot too. At the time, they had no doubt that they'd both be successful in securing a place and would go on to run a heart-warming mother-son marathon that the whole family would be proud of!

At that point, I'd never felt any desire to run myself but I had enjoyed our yearly Sunday morning tradition of watching the marathon together, so I also entered the ballot. Jo and Simon figured "In for a penny…" and made their ballot entries too. Stuart's dad Arthur was the only one who would not even entertain it.

And we were quite confident that all five of us would get a place and run it together as one big happy family.

As it turned out, Stuart was the only one of us that

was successful in the ballot, and even that was lucky. We now realise that to think all five of us would get in on the same attempt was really very naïve; however, to this day Julie, Simon and Jo are all very relieved they didn't get a place in the ballot. Witnessing Stuart's experience on the day was quite enough to put them all off for good. Somehow I wasn't scared off and I did go on to do the London Marathon a few years later, as you know. Stuart and I had very different experiences – I had a great race, achieving a time I was proud of, never hitting the wall and retaining all 10 toenails. I often remind him how successful my first marathon was compared to his.

Back then, Stuart had almost no concept of what running a marathon was like. His only experience, like many of us, was watching the London Marathon coverage from the sofa on a lazy Sunday morning, once a year. Usually with a bacon sandwich and a cuppa. Pretty much as far removed as you could be from actually running a marathon on the streets of London with 40,000 other runners.

It has to be said that the buzz of the television coverage on race day does make you believe you could roll up the following day and crack out a quick 26.2 miles in a tutu, smiling and high-fiving kids, all whilst raising thousands for charity before returning home to rapturous applause and adoration from your friends, family and neighbours!

Stuart was committed to running a marathon approximately seven months from then, and he began his training; his very first run was a lap of the large field near our house. Not yet familiar with the existence of GPS running watches, Stuart estimated this field to be about 2 miles around the perimeter and he felt this would be a good starting point for someone who had never really run or been particularly active since school.

He returned 15 minutes later, gasping for air, and dripping in sweat. That evening, once he regained control of his lungs and his legs stopped shaking, Google Maps informed him that a lap of the field was approximately 600 metres.

Over the next few weeks and months I didn't see Stuart training a whole lot, although there was a lot of talk about it. I didn't really know myself what proper marathon training looked like, so to me one 45-minute run a week may well have been right on target. I know better now, obviously. As does Stuart!

There were some signs of progression towards the end of his training 'plan', however, with one of his best training runs coming a few weeks ahead of race day. I was impressed to hear about the 15-mile out-and-back run between home in Coventry and Kenilworth, a neighbouring town.

"Impressive, running ALL the way to Kenilworth and back!" I said to myself. We had only ever driven it and although not miles away, it seemed like a long enough distance to run. At that point, I certainly wouldn't have considered running there and back.

Much quicker than expected, marathon weekend

arrived. Stuart spent most of it looking pale and feeling queasy. He didn't talk much. Unfortunately for him, he did walk a lot! I thought a sight-seeing day in London on the Saturday would be lovely but I didn't think about the 9 miles we would spend on foot! Well, I didn't need to, did I? I wasn't running a marathon the next day.

Sunday finally arrived and as we left our Air BnB, Stuart looked even paler than he had on Saturday. Although he is not a fan of any public transport on any day of the week, much less London public transport on marathon weekend, we headed for Greenwich via the DLR. Given Stuart's feelings about public transport, and the volume of people on the train, the journey was not the camaraderie-filled experience that some people were enjoying. He was not one of the runners sharing stories of nervousness and excitement with their fellow athletes. He was the runner sitting quietly on the edge of their seat, staring at their feet, and very subtly rocking back and forth!

Arriving at the start zone, Stuart made it very clear that he didn't really want our company and was too nervous to make idle chatter. He just wanted to be left alone with his thoughts so we, his loyal supporters, headed off into London looking for the best place to begin our day of spectating.

We often argue that spectating is the harder task and greater achievement of marathon day and if I recall correctly, Jo and I racked up a total of nine different spectator locations, including the start and finish lines. We really worked hard that day!

One sighting that sticks out in my mind, and actually we have it on video, is from mile 18. It begins with Stuart coming into sight from the left and we all go mad in the foreground, cheering and whooping and calling his name. We are so excited to catch a glimpse of him, relatively close to the end (the end of the race, that is, not his own expiration!).

You can clearly see the moment Stuart spots us (or most likely hears us!). He begins to veer across to the right-hand side of the route where we are positioned, weaving through the other runners – who include Sir Richard Branson dressed as a caterpillar alongside a 34-person butterfly. Our cheers get louder and you can see a number of hands reach out in anticipation of high-fives and hugs as Stuart approaches. He finally reaches us and our excitement peaks.

"This is it! Here he comes!" We are practically giddy!

With a sideways glance towards us and devoid of any emotion, Stuart utters the words: "I hate you, Mum," and carries on running.

We all just stood there, deflated.

"Oh…"

Like many new runners, a big mistake Stuart made during this first London Marathon was doing very little research on running kit. Imagine running a marathon (actually, imagine running any distance) in your old school PE trainers. Imagine wearing old scratchy gym socks with holes in the heels. Well, Stuart wore both these things on race day and, to top off such an inspired sporting look, an England football shirt!

Stuart did buy some shorts for the occasion because he didn't own any previous to the race but other than that, his first race-day kit was made up mainly of his school gym kit from 10 years earlier.

Not being one to engage in 'fast fashion', you can still find Stuart wearing those shorts today. In fact, I believe he's currently out on a training run in said shorts. What's left of them.

You might be wondering about the decision to run in an England football shirt.

As a family, we agreed the England top was a really good idea as red would be so easy to spot. Yes, that's right, we thought a red top would be easy to spot in a crowd of 40,000 runners at the London Marathon. As we discovered, at least 12 charities wear red, at least 10 running clubs wear red and at least 20,000 of the general running public chose to wear red that day. All we could see was a sea of red! As it turns out, we were OK with the Stuart-spotting in the end because he was always preceded by a runner in a full-sized giraffe costume. Yes, as the race went on the gap between them widened, with the giraffe taking a commanding lead, but at least we always knew we hadn't missed Stuart when the giraffe's head popped into view above the hordes of runners.

One thing we found out much later is that

Kenilworth – the location of Stuart's longest and most successful training run – is actually 6 miles away, not the 7.5 that would be required to run a full 15 miles as he had stated. Much later still, Stuart revealed that he hadn't quite reached Kenilworth itself but rather Kenilworth Road. Kenilworth Road does indeed go into Kenilworth but Stuart did not; he reached the start of Kenilworth Road and turned around for a grand total of 3 miles there and 3 miles back. Six miles. His 'best' marathon training run turned out to be 6 miles.

He has never taken marathon training lightly since; however, the damage had been done and from the second he slumped on the floor in Horse Guard's Parade after that first marathon, Simon, Jo and Julie were committed to never entering the ballot again.

Stuart has actually been successful in three further London Marathon ballots to date – either under his own steam or through one of his running or triathlon clubs. Anyone who has wanted to run the London Marathon will likely know that so many runners spend year after year suffering ballot rejections, so you might wonder how he has come to be so successful. There's no explanation; it's just good luck – and it is OK to hate him for this. His three further attempts have all been very successful though and well trained for – he learnt his lesson in no uncertain terms after spending a whole week after that first one coming down the stairs on his bum and barely able to stomach food.

It was one of my own running blunders, however, that started me off on the path to writing this book. This story is one I come back to all the time and I usually can't tell it for laughing. At least now people will be able to read about it and I can just wet myself in the corner! It probably won't translate as funnily in print. It was maybe one of those 'you had to be there' moments but nonetheless it is the story that made me want to start writing down all the stories, so here goes…

One day a few years ago, four of us decided to jump in the car and head out into the countryside for a 10k trail race. It was Sunday, like many races are, and we left early as it was some 20 miles away and none of us had been there before. The early Sunday morning lack of traffic meant we actually arrived in really good time – first ones there, in fact – and we were pleased that we had left ourselves enough time to relax and get race-ready, as we all tend to feel a little anxious on race day.

To me, a 10k trail is not to be underestimated. It can be quite taxing on the legs and you have to pay attention to branches, mud, leaves and so on, all of which can be hazardous. No runner wants a broken leg! Getting there nice and early helped to calm my anxieties a little.

Driving in, we realised that we had arrived so early that the gates to the stately home location were still closed but had been unlocked in preparation for the race. Two of us got out of the car, forced the heavy gates open and held them back while our driver headed in to have their pick of car parking spaces. We spent a little time admiring the grounds and the property itself, taking selfies and chit chatting about our various approaches to the race. Then we realised we probably needed to start warming up… a bit.

We did some basic stretches.

We didn't take it to extremes though, as we are not the kind of runners who are interested in doing a full warm-up routine, no matter how many times we hear it recommended to us. We did a quick quad stretch that really had no benefit at all other than to make us feel like we had ticked off another box on the pre-race checklist.

Time pressed on and I noticed it was after 9:30. The race was due to start at 10 and there wasn't a single soul to be seen, except us four. We'd been busy taking selfies and warming up (!) until now and we hadn't noticed that we were still the only ones there. We all had the same sinking thought at the same time…

"Oh my God, we're at the wrong venue!"

We grabbed our phones, panicking, wondering if we'd have time to get to the correct location. The wishy-washy phone signal out in the sticks didn't help our anxiety. Luckily, after holding her phone up high near a tree for a minute, my brilliant friend Emma was able to get enough signal to decide that we were exactly where we should be.

"Phew!"

Except where was everybody else? Maybe we were panicking over nothing. Do trail runners just casually turn up minutes before the race start? Are they less highly-strung than most other runners?

"Yes, I think I've heard that somewhere," we all agreed. We carried on waiting.

At 09:53 and still no signs of life, once again we found ourselves panicking.

"Wrong day?"

"Wrong time?"

"What is going on?"

This time it was me waving my phone in the air and I was able to get a small amount of signal long enough to go online and check the race timings…

Second and fourth Sunday, January to March, 10am.

We were spot on.

Surely even if no one except us four had signed up to the race, we could at least expect to see a marshal or race director somewhere. We were getting quite angry with the race organisers by this point, mentally preparing the reviews we were going to leave on social media. We checked their social media channels and there were no posts warning of it being cancelled.

It was quite bizarre. I honestly started to doubt if I was even awake. Maybe there was something spooky going on? Had a zombie apocalypse descended while we were en route to the venue and the population of trail runners had been wiped out?

By now, we were not only cross with the organisers

but were also starting to get a little crabby with each other. Despite being good friends, we started to snipe and bicker. It was pretty cold too, being March, and we were very fed up. And confused!

I sat in the back of the car to warm up and read and re-read the details out loud to myself, over and over.

"Every second and fourth Sunday* 10am."

I read it again, slower.

"Every second and fourth Sunday* 10am."

Wait, what does that little star mean?

Turns out it means "Look at the small print, you fucking idiots."

"Every second and fourth Sunday* 10am … *Except in months with five Sundays where it switches to every second and fifth Sunday at 10am."

We were a week early!

Not only that, but we were also trespassing on private property and had been for the last hour. All the very serious 'No trespassing' and 'This is private property' and 'Trespassers will be prosecuted' signs suddenly came sharply into focus as realisation properly sank in that we had made a huge blunder. We hadn't read the race instructions properly.

Not wanting to end up on the news, we hot-footed it to the car at a pace far faster than we would have ever moved in the actual race.

The final straw came as we threw ourselves in to the car, *Dukes of Hazzard* style, and our designated driver sped off, not realising that one of the girls was not quite in the car as fully as she would have liked to be…

Don't worry, she's OK…

…now!

We did not go back the following week. We've never been back since. In fact, the four of us have never organised to go to another race together. What makes me laugh most about our small blunder was the level of cockiness we displayed as we strolled around those stately home grounds like the resident peacocks, pleased as punch with ourselves. Strong independent women, ticking all the boxes for a great race! As it turns out, those strong independent women failed to obey the simplest race-day rule: read the race instructions thoroughly.

We're not the only ones though! I heard from one morbidly embarrassed runner who made a huge cock-up when booking the Birmingham 10k for himself and his partner.

Having done the race before and with six months or so to go, the confirmation email was filed without much attention and training began (not too much training, of course!).

Over the next few months, travel arrangements were made along with plans to meet up with other runners near the start. When race week arrived and other runners started sharing Instagram photos of their bib numbers, it dawned on the husband that theirs hadn't arrived. A quick email to the organisers set his mind at rest: "If it doesn't arrive this week, you can collect a spare from the information tent on race morning."

The bibs never arrived but he was not too concerned and instead they just set off 20 minutes earlier to pick up their spare bibs. Arriving at the information tent, jolly and cheery ahead of a morning's race, they greeted the volunteer with a smile and asked for their replacement bibs. The volunteer scrolled through the list but, to everyone's confusion, was unable to find them.

"Check again, please," he requested.

Scrolling through the list again, the volunteer confirmed: "Your name's not down."

Getting less cheery as time rolled on, the runner pulled his phone out, found the email and waved it under the nose of the volunteer. "See. Can you look into this please and get us some spare bib numbers?"

By his own admission, he was now acting a little smug. Until…

"Sir, that's the Birmingham Alabama 10k. In America."

"Oh…" was all he was able to mutter, as his wife's eyes bore in to the side of his face, steam coming from her ears, blood about to come from his own. He had signed up to the wrong country's 10k and hadn't even noticed. He hadn't noticed the fees had been listed in dollars. He hadn't noticed the date was entirely different. He didn't read his race pack!

And, speaking of husbands who don't read the race pack and find themselves in trouble with their wives, my buddy Daniel shared the following for us to enjoy.

An enchanted fairy-tale set in the fields of the White Star Running Bad Cow weekend. Names have been changed to protect identities, so you will never know if Daniel is sharing someone else's race faux pas or if it was indeed his own...

Race Report
Daniel's Bad Cow Race Weekend

Ladies and gentlemen, the story you are about to read is true. The names are changed to protect the innocent but perhaps in this case the total incompetence of one person really should be highlighted to save future runners! So settle down with a nice cup of tea or a pint of Dorset cider and enjoy this tale of a rather unexpected journey.

Once upon a time there lived a young man and his amazing wife (I had to add that bit in as I am still in the dog house – as you will soon find out!). The husband carefully attended to his wife's heart's desire to join the 100 Marathon Club. Even after she was impaired during a nocturnal marathon attempt less than two years ago and she became the evillest of all evil witches because she couldn't run, he still doted on her.

Over many months our heroic husband coached his wife back to fitness, fitter than ever before. Not only was she able to run marathons again, but her running improved beyond her wildest dreams; his coaching was so good she PB'd at every distance over the year!

#coachandhusbandoftheyear

Booking her 19th marathon for her, he chose carefully and opted for a weekend away in Dorset with White Star Running, whose hoodies and T-shirts proclaim them to be fine purveyors of races (or nutty races for nutty people, depending on which piece of merchandise you select).

The Bad Cow weekend offered a range of races over the two days: The Bad Cow Frolic on Saturday (a 12-hour race in which you run as many laps as you can in the time allowed), and a choice between a marathon or half marathon on the Sunday. The husband signed them both up for the Sunday marathon.

After managing a double marathon a few weeks earlier and having already paid for a weekend of camping, the husband quickly checked to see if there were spaces on the Saturday Frolic on the off chance he could make it a cheeky double marathon weekend. Alas, the Frolic was full and he had to accept that just the Sunday marathon would suffice.

Soon enough, race weekend came around and the children were left with their grandfather on the Friday evening. The husband carefully packed the car full of everything needed for a successful running weekend, in order that the following morning's alarm call could be delayed until the last possible moment so his gorgeous wife (has my flattery bordered into obsequiousness?) could get a few extra minutes of beauty sleep – although totally unneeded.

As we all know, Saturday is really parkrunday, and so it was for our happy couple. After a liquid porridge breakfast (think gritty baby food), the drive south for the weekend's marathon took them to Newbury parkrun. Despite an invading hoard of orcs to avoid en route (OK, an American Army re-enactment group complete with tanks and a jerk chicken van), the parkrun course was flat and had pacers, so in the end, a faster parkrun than planned was run. Once over, the journey to Dorset continued in good time and our couple arrived just after 12 noon, feeling parkrun fresh. The Saturday Frolic was already underway.

Their tent was erected with speed and style and so it was that the cunning husband headed over to the race administration tent to find out where the showers were and collect their race numbers for Sunday. This meant that the remains of the day could be spent lavishing attention on his dazzling better half – a trip to Corfe Castle, a delicious cream tea, a seaside stroll and a pre-marathon pizza.

But wait…

SHOCK HORROR! Both husband and wife were missing from the list of participants for the marathon; they weren't even down for the half marathon in error.

Retaining an air of calm akin to that of a Californian surfer dude, the husband said, "There must be a mistake," and consulted his emails to find out how this error had occurred. The helpful Gemma at White Star Running began hunting down the entries online.

Just as motorways haven't reached Dorset yet, nor has decent 4G or 3G or actually any G mobile phone signal. So the husband and Gemma both circled the field outside the administration tent, devices held skywards, carefully avoiding the Frolic runners, who were currently racing.

"Oh. I am/you are booked onto the Frolic!" said

both husband and Gemma in unison.

The Frolic that is already underway. Not tomorrow's marathon.

Glancing down at his Garmin and seeing that the hour digits still included a 12 (OK, it was 12:54), the husband exclaimed, "So we still have time to run a marathon today if we start right now!"

Quickly, Gemma sorted out their race numbers.

Running back to the car, the husband stripped off his cotton traveling shirt (much like Superman he felt) and found the plastic bag with that morning's parkrun T-shirt inside. With a quick wringing to remove the worst of the sweat, the damp purple volunteers T-shirt was back on. He slipped out of his driving shoes and into his old faithful elasticated laced road shoes, also moist from parkrun, and chirped, "I'm ready, let's go!"

The wife ditched her warm hoody and grabbed her parkrun waist pack so she at least had her inhalers and phone and the couple jogged to the start in the afternoon sunshine. Across the timing mat they travelled, beginning the first of the six laps required to run a marathon.

As soon as the couple left the safety of the first field and entered the woods, the wife's moans and complaints were directed right at the poor husband. His poor organisation! How could someone muck up the day they are due to run a marathon?

Given the late start, their pace slowly crept up as they had to make sure they made the cut off time. The major advantage of the increase in pace was that the wife's whinging was replaced by gasping.

The course wound its way around pretty rural areas, up gentle slopes (after previously doing their other events, the Invader and East Farm, these slopes couldn't be described as hills in White Star Running terms), along fern-lined paths, through woodland and along farm tracks. Despite the sandy hills (complete with sandcastles made during the race by runners!), the dry conditions, compacted gravel and small road section made road shoes seem a sensible choice.

As lap two started, the weather changed. Just like the overall mood of the weekend, gone went the sunshine and down came dark clouds, followed by the first of many showers of heavy rain. For one of the parties, the rain came as a delight; to the other, it brought further discomfort. An already moist shirt became saturated and shivers began.

And so it was at lap two that our couple separated. (Not maritally; just for the remainder of the race.) One left to go back to the tent to put on fresh, clean, dry kit and find a running jacket. The other ran on! The poor husband realised that if he stopped running this soon he wouldn't want to restart.

The joy of a White Star Running race is the Lovestation – an aid station that offers trail runners their stomachs' wildest desires! Not gels, but tasty real food treats and alcohol. Due to the lack of pre-race fuelling, this gazebo became paradise. A few cocktail sausages, a Scotch egg, a slice or two of watermelon all washed down with a plastic cup or two of not flat-enough coke became the necessary sustenance for these marathon runners.

Rain changes a course and so it was that the heavy showers replaced the sandy slopes with slippery, muddy ravines. Suddenly, trail shoes (even better, mud claws) seemed more the order of the day. But stopping just for a change of shoes was completely ignored by our now forlorn husband. What was allowed was a decent stoppage at the superb portaloos (think of the cleanest race portaloo you have ever used and these are far better!). This was certainly necessary as the normal pre-race ablutions had been completely forgotten in the rush to start the race. Yes, this may seem like time wasted, but the husband wasn't wearing a buff so a stop in the woods near the roaming cows, albeit likely to be quicker than queuing for a portaloo, had to be ruled out.

On the fourth visit to the aid station, the volunteers commented to the bedraggled husband that they felt sorry for him. At first, he thought this was because they knew about his small mistake with the race dates and how that had led to a very disgruntled wife. A wife that he had then deserted mid-race. But no, it was because of his nipples. Two large bloody circles had appeared on his shirt – and for blood to show up through the damp purple colour meant there was a lot of it.

At this point though, the husband was ambivalent to any self-harm and he ran on, telling them it was fine!

Another 4.4 miles of thinking about and feeling every slight movement of his shirt meant that at the next visit to the Lovestation, the offer of nipple lubrication was graciously accepted. This really went above and beyond the normal duty of a supporter hug or a kiss that the Lovestation lovelies usually offer to power runners on their way for their remaining miles.

Raising his shirt to receive the lubrication elicited gasps from the volunteers – unfortunately not of lust for the Adonis-like chest of the husband, but because of the shredded, bloody state of his nipples. A full self-adhesive dressing was applied, followed by tape to secure it to his moist hairy chest!

This delay allowed the long-suffering wife to come into view on the horizon. After briefly considering running off (especially after hearing that suggestions had been made to the wife regarding where a husband's battered body could be left unnoticed for many weeks!), the husband stayed and waited for his first wife (well, after experiences like this, things could end in divorce!) so he could run the last 6-ish miles with her.

However, despite his good intentions, it was not to be. Not because of his wife's anger at him – the 11 beautiful miles alone had eased that and she was buoyed by the increased confidence that a lap under head torch would be unnecessary – but because of the differing pace. The variability of weather over the multiple laps (sun, rain, cold rain, sun, rain, drizzle, cool evening) meant that for the wife, a deliberate decision had been taken to slow down on the final lap to take pictures and give her asthmatic lungs the chance to recover before next week's marathon. The husband, however, when walking, looked soon to depart this world, as he staggered along painfully. When running, he was far more relaxed and at ease. So it was at the arrival of the first incline that our couple again parted ways, this time as friends, to meet very soon at the finish.

Later, the wife's eyes sparkled more than the medal she was wearing around her neck as she contemplated the compensation she would extract from her husband for his foolish error. Or maybe it was the malevolent delight of having to help remove the taped-on dressing from his chest hair!

The next day, the couple clapped the marathon runners off on their race; the race they should have been doing, had things gone to plan. The wife, dressed in her new pink White Star Running rugby shirt, brushed away the remains of a delicious breakfast from her husband's chin and commented that White Star Running really do put on great races and that more runners should give them a go. Just on the right day!

Chapter Six
Sorry For What I Said
During My Bad Run!

Amongst our running bubble (a collective noun for us that we didn't know existed until the COVID-19 pandemic but that fits our running group perfectly) it is not uncommon to receive an apologetic WhatsApp message shortly after a race or training session together, along the lines of:

"Sorry for what I said during that run."

"Obviously you are *not* a treacherous bitch with sadistic tendencies and a thirst for the spilled blood of your fellow runners."

"I was just a bit hungry."

It's called runner's rage and I am afflicted by it. When I start to get tired or overwhelmed on a long run (actually, let's be honest, even on a short run), I get snappy, irritated and agitated. I'm sure you can go and read all about the hormones and emotions that are involved and why this occurs, but you definitely do know by now that this book is not designed to explain what happens, scientifically, when running. Quite frankly, even if I knew about the science involved and how I could manage my emotions mid-run, I'm too lazy to do anything different and I'd still be snapping people's heads off on my runs, then apologising afterwards. And I know my friends would too. We're all OK with it.

The worst bit is that sometimes my rage is directed at inanimate objects, sometimes even just the weather. In hindsight, the following is a funny story; however, at the time, it was pretty horrible and probably needed addressing clinically.

I was at roughly mile 11 of a 15-mile marathon training run and it was going terribly. My legs had that feeling we all know too well – that running through treacle feeling – and my lungs were burning. I was hurting everywhere.

That all makes it sound like I was running fast, doesn't it?

I wasn't!

It had been particularly windy during the entirety of my run but what I noticed was that no matter what direction I'd been running, the wind always felt like it was coming at me head on.

What are the chances that the wind changed direction every time I did?

I was running (slowly!) through one of my local parks and I remember starting to grumble to myself, muttering about the "bloody wind" and finding myself more and more frustrated with each step.

If someone else was telling me this story I would be interrupting at this point to ask, "Why didn't you just stop?"

I should have stopped the run for my own mental, physical and emotional wellbeing. I was hating every minute of it but I felt so much runner's guilt at the thought of quitting my run, even though I shouldn't – but, as you know, sometimes I practise what I preach and sometimes I don't.

I am but a runner!

And there are lots of quotes on mugs and T-shirts that perpetuate this need to never give up. They talk about personal strength, challenging yourself, beating the people on the sofa, putting one foot in front of the other, finding your inner strength, never giving up, running with your heart when your legs stop. Plus there's Strava and social media to contend with and the knowledge that everyone will see your 'failed' attempt.

I do very strongly believe that if it wasn't for social media, we runners would be far kinder to ourselves. I see runners putting themselves through the mill on days they really shouldn't and I always wonder whether they still would have done it if the internet was scrapped and no one would ever know they'd given it a miss. Just before I get back to my windy day story, I feel like I should finish this digressive paragraph with a heart-felt, inspirational statement:

"Run what's right for you. If needs be, let your body heal and be stronger next time."

But I'm never going to do that myself, so I can't in good conscience preach it to others!

And you wouldn't listen anyway.

Just forget I said it!

Anyway, back to the wind. It eventually got too

much for me and, mid-run, I looked up (why up?) and screamed very much out loud: "Fuck you, wind, just fuck off!" Then I started to cry.

So did the children of the family who witnessed my outburst.

I ran on (and so did the family; they just went in the other direction).

I was plodding away, legs heavy, chest on fire, tears, shame, guilt, my internal monologue going crazy.

I know you know what I'm talking about.

Another mile or two further along, I finally gave up/let myself have a rest break and stopped to sit on the wall of a car dealership. (It was Hyundai, for the car buffs reading this.)

I ended up sitting there for 10 minutes contemplating my bad choices during the run and my expletive outburst. It's a shame I can't send the statutory "I'm sorry" WhatsApp to the family I scared.

I finally realised that I might have been wrong to push myself so hard when I clearly needed a rest. I felt so good getting that clarity and understanding of what I had done wrong and how to protect myself next time. Lesson learnt!

I got up off the wall and proceeded to run the long way home, so maybe it wasn't quite lesson learnt but I got a little closer to being a more mature, mindful runner. Until the next time I went out and did the same thing over again…

I am not the worst rager out there, however, and if

there was an award for mid-run potty mouth, it would go to Jo. Hands down. And she would gladly accept the award with pride and joy.

Mid-run, Jo gets consumed by her inner running demon and becomes a foul-mouthed lout (said with love!). She once told a kindly photographer to "Fuck off with that thing" in the final steps of a race. To be fair, he did shout "Well done!" so I don't know how else she could have responded.

She even told me to "Fuck off with that thing" once when I was standing injured at the side of a race taking photos and supporting.

Jo is not to be judged for her outbursts and indeed, in the safety of our running bubble, we all respect each other's need to let off steam. Recently Jo texted me, asking if I would go running with her on an evening where she'd just about had enough of the world and all its people. I was in a similar emotional state, snapping at inanimate objects around my house and sending strongly worded emails to organisations who had 'wronged me'. I gladly accepted her offer and we hit the streets for a little over 5k, which went by in a flash as we took turns ranting and raving about our problems without ever really thinking about the running. Neither of us had fancied our normal club training session that night, simply because it is usually full of happy, encouraging, lovely people and we needed to moan and whine. Had we gone to regularly scheduled training we would have either brought down the other runners, which wouldn't have been fair, or they would have perked us up, which was not what we wanted! We wanted to turn the air blue and enjoy the relief you feel when you finally get things off your chest. We were rage running!

Rage is not the only emotion that comes to the surface through running, however – there's a whole range of emotions it stirs up. I have cried on many runs, both happy and sad tears, for many reasons. Once, when I was suffering from unexplained anxiety (that a cognitive behaviour therapist later unearthed to be related to training for my first marathon – Liverpool marathon, which I ultimately failed to achieve), I cried for no reason mid-run. I literally couldn't explain it to the kind runners who kept asking if I was OK. I didn't even know if they were happy or sad tears; they just came on during a set of hill reps and wouldn't stop.

One of my favourite happy tears moments was when I once came dead last in a run.

Technically, I've been last place in a few races but where there were other runners who were listed in the results tables as DNS (did not start), so technically I still beat them, right? No?

My genuinely very last place was at my running club's handicap race and I was favoured with quite a generous handicap, being the slow runner I am. To still come last despite this was a real shitshow. I clearly didn't just run my normal level of crapness; I levelled up. The final runner set off more than half an hour after me and still flew past me a hundred metres before the end. I remember hearing him coming up behind me as I tried to eke out any last bit of energy I had to keep him at bay, but it wasn't enough.

My dad always tells me (and I would happily, genuinely tell OTHER runners), "Someone has to come last," but as I was endlessly passed by runner after runner, all of whom had set off after me, those words meant nothing. I didn't want to be the someone, especially as my body had feelings more akin to running really fast than really slow. Surely the aches, pains, sweat, huffing and puffing were signs of me giving it my all? How was I still nothing more than an obstacle for the later runners to hurdle over?

It doesn't matter what we tell ourselves, or others. No one sets out to come last and I'm sure we all secretly like to 'beat' at least one other person. As a runner, I have said a thousand times, "Don't worry about coming last, just enjoy it," and I've said two thousand times, "Oh well, at least I didn't come last."

The fickle nature of runners, me in particular, rears its ugly head again!

I'm not sure I believe most runners when they say they truly don't care if they come last. Mostly because I've heard a lot of people talk about how it's the taking part that counts – before sharing their race position and how happy they are with it in their post-race Facebook post. If they didn't care about finish positions, why did they even mention theirs? It's made me a bit cynical! Plus, if we are all so OK with coming last, why is there a tail-person at parkrun to ensure no one else is last? I think we just have to admit the uncomfortable truth: no one really wants to be last. It doesn't make you judgemental of the person who does come last, it's just a weird running paradox. It's maybe a bit of a running NIMBY phenomenon. It's totally OK for someone to be last, just not me!

One great thing about this emotional side of running is that it brings out our inner strengths. Despite my feelings during the handicap race, I carried on to the bitter end and found waiting for me at the finish line a large crowd of finished runners cheering me in. We get great support and cheers in all our club races; however, on this occasion it was on a scale far beyond what you get when you finish mid-pack, which is where I am often found. I felt a lovely sense of support and friendship having everyone cheering me on.

I still didn't want to be last though – I absolutely would have traded all the support and kindness for placing further up the table and securing some points towards the overall trophy. (I had won the trophy once in a previous season and letting the title go was hard!) I guess it is OK to be disappointed with your time or finish place, even if you got a lot of cheers. This, of course, is just a reflection of where I am now with my running. I know what I can do, so coming last isn't up to my own personal standards. I'm reminded of Sir Mo Farah's interview after his 'rubbish' attempt at the London Marathon 2019, where he commented that he was disappointed with himself for placing fifth. Imagine being disappointed with fifth place?! But we all have a goal – and if we don't meet that goal, it is disappointing. If your goal is to get out and run, and you spend all day stuck indoors, you will feel disappointed.

It's the same when you know you can finish at the front but end up last – you had a goal, you tried to get there and you didn't achieve it. I think it's totally OK to miss goals but it doesn't mean you have to be happy about it. Being a runner doesn't mean you have to always be positive and smiling and acting like it's the best thing ever. You can be pissed off with running and it won't make you less of a runner!

Interestingly, in that same race where Mo came fifth, a runner named Lukas Bates was foiled in his Guinness World Record attempt to complete the fastest time while dressed as a landmark. Dressed as Big Ben and looking to me like a very competent 'serious' runner, he found that he couldn't cross the finish line as the height of the costume exceeded the height of the finish line arch! This is one of the reasons I wanted to write this book. I felt there was a distinct lack of literature that raised the real issues of runners such as the need to measure the height of your costume before race day.

Most runners at some point will feel the sting of marathon ballot rejections. Occasionally, there is relief that you didn't get in (mostly when you only signed up to the race because you were drunk) and there's always one runner in your circle of running friends who acts like a race pimp and takes a slightly shady approach to 'encouraging' you into races you never would consider. They usually do this when you are drunk at a running party and easy prey. That's how I ended up taking part in races like the Thunder Run (a 24-hour race with continuous 10k relay legs), the Hilly 100, and Las Vegas half marathon (to be fair, that last one I didn't need quite as much persuading). But back to the frustration of marathon rejections…

More often than not a ballot rejection hurts – and none more so, it seems, than the London Marathon. I think what makes it particularly tricky is the fact that some people get in time and time again (like Stuart) whilst others get a place and fritter it away. All the while there are runners who have never had the luck to get in just once. I've applied seven times and never been lucky in the ballot. I did get lucky in our club ballot one year (London Marathon gives away a certain number of places to clubs registered with British Athletics, the exact amount dependent on membership numbers). I distinctly remember my raffle ticket number, 147, and it was pulled out fourth, the last of the club places we had for that year. I was ecstatic!

Unfortunately, my joy was short-lived. What the club hadn't realised was that this particular year the boundaries changed and the number of places allocated was reduced. Our club membership size meant we were no longer entitled to four, but three places. I was last in and first out! I don't think our club committee has ever drawn that ballot since without having the exact number of places written in blood by the London Marathon organisers. I was gutted but I understood. Some of my angrier-natured, fiery friends told me I should demand a new club ballot or demand I get the first place in next year's ballot. I understand they were just trying to support and soothe me but I would never do that. It would only create frustration and disappointment for someone else in the club. I sucked it up and I got my turn eventually (you haven't forgotten I ran a marathon, have you?!) via a charity place, so I'm not bitter.

The most London Marathon rejections I have heard about came from my very funny, very down-to-earth clubmate Jonathan. Throughout his long running career he had over 20 rejections before he was finally successful with a Good For Age place and ran the October 2022 incarnation of the event. (It reverts back to being held in April as of 2023.) Jonathan is currently training with, and ran the marathon with, a hitchhiker named Trevor. Said hitchhiker happens to be a brain tumour. It is impressive and humbling, the strength and determination it must take to tackle a marathon in the midst of such a life-changing condition. Jonathan, I'm sure, would disagree, being the down-to-earth, just-get-on-with-it runner that he is, but I am still in awe. Particularly so as he also raised almost £2,500 for the Brain Tumour Charity whilst training for and running the marathon.

I know there is a fair amount of frustration at the way the London Marathon ballot is conducted and how this results in multiple, sometimes life-long rejections for so many. Some runners believe you should only get one attempt and once you've had a ballot place you are out of the running, at least for X number of years. Others feel that only runners of a certain ability should get in, proving themselves in earlier races before they can apply. Some feel that the charity, Good For Age, club and celebrity places should be reduced. Some feel that a place should be automatically available after a certain number of rejections (a system that used to be in place but which is no longer sustainable, based on capacity).

I have to say, I don't agree. It probably seems very easy for me to say that, having run the London Marathon, but I promise you I felt this way beforehand too. Having experienced the joy for myself, I want everyone who wants to do it to have their chance to experience it but unfortunately, even with my limited knowledge of organising a world-leading marathon, I know it's not possible. What makes this race so special and cements it as the race so many runners desperately want to do is the essence of the ballot – that anyone could do it, even if that means some do it more than once. That person who was successful last year may have had the race from hell, so I can't begrudge them another attempt. The charities, the celebrities, the runners who have never run before but make it their mission to complete this particular race, is where its glory lies.

The charities are responsible for some of the biggest entertainment highlights on the course. The Elite and Good For Age runners put on a competitive show that we are all excited to witness. The everyday real-life runners bring out the costumes, the noise and the heart-warming stories of overcoming tragedy and adversity. The club runners fly the flag for grassroots running. London Marathon has a colossal sense of community spirit and this brings out the masses of spectators, even those who have no interest in running but just come out to watch this wonderful spectacle. If you take all this away to allow more general ballot places, it becomes just another marathon in a big city, of which there are plenty. It sucks, and I feel for anyone who has faced years of rejection, but if it changed from what it currently is, I just don't think it would be the London Marathon we all want to run.

If you're waiting patiently for your turn to run the London Marathon, I hope you get your chance soon. When the time comes, be prepared to ride a rollercoaster of emotions, from excitement to fear to joy to exhaustion. You're going to love it!

When I was reading through the various race reports that were submitted to me for this book, one stood out as particularly indicative of the emotions runners go through in a race; it came from my very kind, lovely friend Elaine. It's also about the London Marathon, so this is one of those chapters where I feel I've absolutely nailed the link between the chapter content and the race report.

Race Report
Elaine's London Marathon

My friend Katy and I arrived at my sister's house on Friday evening full of beans and very excited – and we didn't go to bed as early as we were supposed to.

I woke the next morning very early but managed to get back to sleep until around 7am. Breakfast was eaten and we were ready for the expo, at which we arrived just before 10am, slightly later than hoped. I couldn't believe how many people were already there and within two hours the place was packed.

I had the biggest grin on my face when I collected my race number and I don't think the grin left until Sunday evening when I was just plain tired.

An hour after we arrived we were still in the Adidas area, mainly because Katy and my sister Angela had their gait analysed, following which Katy purchased the Adidas Boost VMLM‡ trainers (jealous much!). After this, we went straight to my charity stand (Pancreatic Cancer) and said hi again (I had already met them at the Brighton Marathon), shared hugs and wrote some messages for lost loved ones on their message board, which was very emotional.

Next it was free time – and boy, did we make the most of it. We didn't leave until 1:30pm. I never thought I could spend so much time in an expo but the place is absolutely huge! A pair of new seamless

---

‡ Virgin Money London Marathon

running pants bought for £16 (hope they're worth it) and then we headed off to Westfield shopping centre for some much-needed carb loading. Pizza, anyone?

Sunday arrived much sooner than we thought (thank goodness, in a way). I woke at 5:30am for the first job of the day – a trip to the toilet! The second job of the day was to apply a Run Mummy Run tattoo – easy! Next up was to double-check everything, make porridge and generally potter around until it was time to leave at 6:40. Off we went to catch the tube. We were crammed in like sardines but we managed to get a seat in the very last carriage and away we went. The train got fuller and fuller the nearer we got to Blackheath, which meant there was never any doubt that we'd find the start – we just followed everybody else!

Fifteen minutes later and we were well and truly there. It didn't take us very long at all to find the Lucozade stand and the other Run Mummy Run ladies. This is an online community of over 190,000 women who are passionate about running. We support, motivate and empower each other to be active and improve our running skills. There were lots of hugs, kisses and greetings and I got to meet Becky, who was also running for Pancreatic Cancer.

We had a photo op, toilet visit, baggage drop, another toilet visit (and we were freezing by then) and before we knew it, we were making our way to gate 9.

AWAY WE GO!!

It seemed to take forever to actually get to the start line but as we crossed it, I remember saying: "Hey ladies, we're actually running the London Marathon!" It was the best feeling ever (well, almost!).

The first couple of miles consisted of lots of speed bumps and, as you do, every time we ran across one we shouted "HUMP!" (For anybody who runs Kingsbury Water parkrun, you'll often hear this there too!)

The support en route was just incredible. So many people lined the streets to cheer us on, shouting our names. It really was just incredible. By mile 3, the red start runners were on the other side of the road and they joined us around mile 4 – at which point I saw something large up ahead.

"Is that a dinosaur?" I asked.

It was, and as I overtook him I realised it was a gentleman in a T-Rex costume. It was so huge the poor guy ended up ditching his costume at mile 8 as he was injured. Hats off to him; he was brilliant.

Passing the Cutty Sark around mile 6 was awesome but within seconds it was gone again. (That reminds me – where were the awful cobbles people talk about?) Time and people seemed to whizz past and before we knew it we were at mile 10 in 1 hour 50 minutes, which is my fastest 10 miles ever (I am normally 1 hour 55 minutes). We were sailing along quite nicely and the weather couldn't have been better; a lovely cool breeze every now and again.

Mile 12 and as we were approaching Tower Bridge, poor Katy was really starting to struggle and I felt so bad for her. I can't remember much about Tower

Bridge as I was too busy looking for my sister Angela. I do remember seeing the Pancreatic Cancer cheering squad just over the bridge on the left – YAY!

Around the corner, I heard my name being shouted. It was my sister, who was on the corner, but she was behind loads of people and we couldn't get to each other. This is where I became hysterical: "It's my sister and she can't get through. Let her through, let her through!" I cried.

The crowd were great and they let her through. I almost tripped over the barriers getting to her. I dropped my running bottle as we threw our arms around each other and we cried. She asked if I was OK and I said, "Yes, absolutely fine," and I was! I left her and carried on and caught up with Katy and Becky again. At this point Becky (the youngster) carried on ahead and that was the last I saw of her until the Pancreatic Cancer meet up at the end.

Around this point, we passed the 'halfway party', which was very noisy but gave us much needed music and cheers.

We reached mile 15 and there was my sister again. Katy carried on while I stopped for a hug. When I caught up with Katy again I could see she was struggling with pain but we kept on going. I would run on ahead then walk until Katy caught me up. It was at this point that I struggled with my first electrolyte refill. Never put the water in the bottle first… BIG mistake! I looked like I had cocaine all over my hands and bottle. Such a mess!

At mile 17, there was my sister again! This time Katy also received a much-needed hug and on we plodded.

At mile 18, it was time to think about another bottle of electrolytes; powder in first this time! As we approached mile 19 I kept reminding Katy that the Run Mummy Run ladies and our friend Alison would be there and that every time we crossed the tracking pads they would know we were getting closer.

Mile 18.75 (or thereabouts), I spotted Alison and screamed her name. I turned to Katy and screamed: "It's Alison!" and we sprinted for the ladies. OMG, I've never been so happy (well, maybe when my children were born) and there were lots of hugs and kisses with the amazing Run Mummy Run ladies: Alison, Leanne, Shona, Kelly and Shelley. Our friend Anne-Marie joined us too with her selfie stick (a brilliant idea) and then it was time to go (we really didn't want to go).

A bit further on and there was my sister again! Another hug and off we went. Our pace had really slowed down by this point but we plodded on and on.

The Tower of London, 21 miles, and once more there was my sister. Had she been cloned? Another quick hug and goodbye. When will we see her again?

A bit further on, I grabbed a Lucozade gel at the aid station as I was feeling a bit desperate and didn't want to dig into my belt for anything as it might look like a cocaine addict had left their stuff behind! The gel tasted disgusting but it would do. I walked for a while so Katy could catch up and I took the opportunity to text my daughter to see exactly where she was; she was between 24 and 25 miles, just before the London Eye. When I got there, I slowed right down and started looking for her as I didn't want to miss that one opportunity to see my little girl (who was almost 15 at the time and towered over me, but she'll always be my little girl). The poor woman next to me clearly thought I was mental as I was frantically searching the crowd for my daughter. Just as I was explaining what I was doing, I spotted my girl and sprinted over to her for a quick hug and chat before Katy and I headed off again.

Before long, we approached Parliament and, just like that, we turned the right-hand corner and had just 1 mile to go. By now I was walking, albeit at a fast pace (I have short legs, they can move fast!). I gave lots of encouragement to Katy, letting her know that we could do this and how close we were to the finish line.

As we approached The Mall we saw a photographer, so it was JAZZ HANDS! Katy looked at the time and we'd been running 5 hours 58 minutes and 20 seconds. She wanted to finish in under 6 hours and I pointed out that we'd have to go faster as there was still about 100 metres to go. That was all the encouragement Katy needed and before I knew it, we were sprinting! We finished hand in hand in 5 hours 58 minutes and 44 seconds.

All I can say now is bring on the next London Marathon!

Wait for it… I'm not finished.

The finishers' medal area was up ahead and we were desperately looking for Tarnya, our friend from Run Mummy Run. Katy spotted her but as we headed in her direction, another volunteer was handing out medals. "Sorry, but can you not give me my medal?" I asked. "Our friend is just behind you and we really want her to give us our medals."

Thanks Tarnya. I can't tell you what it meant having our medals given to us by another Run Mummy Run lady.

Chapter Seven
The Good...

One of the fun things about being a runner is the banter and camaraderie we have with each other. This becomes most evident during a big race, when the comedy signs of support come out. I asked my running friends to share the best ones they've seen, so if you ever need inspiration to create your own sign to support a runner in your life, please take your pick.

- You're running better than the government!
- Hurry up, we're cold!
- Stuart, we're here!

This was one of my own signs, with a big arrow pointing to where we were standing. It's hard to spot your runner in a big race so let them do the hard work and spot you instead!

- Follow a nice bum!

Also mine, complete with an accurately drawn anatomical diagram

- Smile, you paid to do this!

This was Jo's A-side sign – she made a reversible 2-in-1 sign because she is tenacious!

- Keep Calm and Don't Be Shit!

This was Jo's B-side - the 'Be' was strategically placed so it could also be read as 'Keep Calm and Don't Shit!'

- Run like you stole something!

- 23 miles until you can have a social life again!
- Run like your mum just used your full name!
- This is a lot of work for a free banana!
- Hurry up, this is boring!
- My arms hurt!
- This is an Inspirational Marathon Sign!
- Touch here for power!

(Top tip from me… If there appears to be a hole cut out of the sign, DO NOT TOUCH THERE!)

- Is that a gel in your pocket or are you just pleased to see me?
- Don't stop, people are watching!
- Is this your sister next to me? She's really loud!
- Keep going, random stranger called Dave!

Statistically, a Dave will run past you every four seconds. Probably.

- This parade sucks!
- Nearly finished! #fakenews

During my own biggest race, the London Marathon, I recall touching almost every 'Touch here for power' sign along the way (not the ones with holes cut in them). The spectators had gone to so much trouble to create an exciting, supportive atmosphere, it felt like the least I could do. I might have been running for five hours but they were standing around for five hours, and if they were unlucky they were probably standing right next to another runner's noisy sister! If you ever find yourself standing next to Stuart's sister (i.e. Jo) at a big race, expect to be bleeding from the ears by the end of the day. Jo's cheering skills are second to none, especially when she brings her cow bells!

One of the most heart-warming things about running is the support-lined streets, with people cheering on at races, and that is possibly most evident in the UK at the London Marathon.

This is your regularly-scheduled reminder that I have run the London Marathon…

I've mentioned it so many times now that I'm sure you want me to expand on my experience. It was truly the best day of my running life. Having failed to reach the start line of the Liverpool Marathon a year earlier through a combination of illness and a training schedule that put me under too much pressure, this time I had been more sensible with my training. Instead of taking a 'stock' training plan off the internet that didn't work for me as a person or a runner, I devised my own that fit around my schedule, abilities and goals. This time, I was far less stressed, training was never a chore, and with three weeks to go until race-day, I felt calm and confident. At three days to go, however, I suddenly turned into a bag of nerves – despite training well, I had all the normal fears of any runner facing a new challenge. Would I finish? Would I be last? Would I die? I am not being flippant with that last one; running a marathon can take its toll on your body, particularly if you have any underlying health issues, and I was worried I would keel over. Sadly, it does happen in many races and my sympathies go out to the runners, families and friends who have experienced such sadness at what should be a happy time.

All my fears manifested in pre-race anxiety. I had the jitters, I was nauseous, I was catastrophising and I experienced a whirlwind of emotions, which, collectively, brought on new fear. Would I even get to the start line? Would I freeze in the bedroom of the Air BnB and not be able to walk out of the door, let alone run 26.2 miles?

On the Friday, a few hours before I was due to travel down to London, I was too jittery to relax, so I washed my car. It is the one and only time in my life that I have washed my car. It took me three hours! Saturday, I tried really hard to enjoy the expo. It was a good event with lots to see, do, learn and purchase but I couldn't concentrate – I just needed it to be Sunday morning and I wanted to block out everything up until that point! I was beginning to understand how Stuart felt at his first London Marathon when he just wanted to be left alone and not speak to anyone.

When Sunday finally arrived, my nervousness eased unexpectedly. It must have been just the anticipation of getting to race morning. I was able to eat my much-loved, if not entirely nutritious, pre-race pancakes and I headed to Greenwich Park, where I found the red start entirely calm despite the thousands of runners milling around. You could hear a pin drop! Nervous energy perhaps? Everyone I spoke to seemed to relax as soon as they heard that someone else was nervous. There was a sense of safety in numbers.

And then, all of a sudden... well, after hours of queuing and shuffling...

"I'm running the London Marathon!"

The nerves melted away and I loved it immediately!

During the early miles, running with my friend Kelvin and comforted knowing he had extensive marathon experience, I paced each mile sensibly. I thought about the race ahead and imagined what it would be like to reach Tower Bridge and pass the halfway mark shortly after. I knew at that point I'd be able to start counting down the miles to the end! I knew Jo and some of the family would be at mile 11. I could hear her (and her cow bells) from about mile 10!

The middle miles passed in a blur of noise from the thousands of spectators clapping, shouting and high-fiving! I kept running, which was one of my goals, but it wasn't always easy. I tired, my legs got heavy and every now and then I wished for just a minute of peace from all the noise, but thankfully I never hit the dreaded 'wall' other runners speak of: the completely overwhelming feeling, either physically or mentally, that you cannot run one single step further. One runner suddenly burst into tears beside me, with no warning. I didn't know what to do but she carried on running regardless, just with tears streaming down her face. As you'd expect, I'd been given lots of advice from my running-club friends and one piece in particular stood out. My good pal Paul had told me to just keep visualising finishing the race and what that would feel like. It was a really top tip and it worked well in the harder sections of the race to take my mind off what I was feeling in the moment. I knew Stuart and his mum Julie were in the grandstand and I kept imagining how I'd greet them when mile 26.2 finally arrived.

The first time I felt close to the finish and the first time I really wanted to have a break and walk coincided with one another. I was on Embankment, approaching mile 25 and flagging. The spectators really don't want you to stop running though, and I'm sure they could see it in my face and body language every time I considered it! I fondly remember some of the wonderful things they were shouting. Not just "Go, Jen!" (my name was on my vest) but real words of encouragement from the heart and, as much as I might have glared at the ones shouting: "Don't walk!" I have to be grateful, as running the whole race was one of my main goals.

When I finally saw the '385 yards to go' sign, I stopped for the briefest second to take it all in, as did a runner beside me. We both wanted one last moment before turning the corner onto The Mall, just to appreciate what it had taken to get to this point, and to clear our heads ready to enjoy the buzz of the finish line. After turning that last corner, I spotted Stuart and Julie in the finish stands and I threw my hands in the air, did a little jig and shouted towards them, "I've just run the London Marathon!"

At this point, I need to apologise to Stuart, now I have the knowledge of what a marathon entails...

I apologise for making you walk all around London the day before your first marathon. Especially when you were already underprepared (even though that bit is kinda your fault!).

I now realise that Marathon Eve is for relaxing (or at least fighting the anxiety!) and carb-loading – which, if you've done it by the book, you'll have begun a good few weeks beforehand, making nutrition an integral part of your training. If you're like me, however, and you're not a by-the-book runner, you will have eaten a few bowls of pasta and maybe a baked potato the week before (it will all have been white pasta and white potatoes, of course!) and now, on the eve of the marathon, you will be cramming in bowlfuls of creamy, garlicky pasta and dough balls followed by tiramisu and coffee (can you guess my go-to pre-race restaurant?) and telling yourself it's carb-loading.

While reading up about the London Marathon, I found some interesting facts on the BBC Sports Get Inspired website that I think the average reader of this book would enjoy[§].

- On average, running a marathon will cause you to burn calories worth 10.5 burgers. That's about 2,600 calories.

In my mind, those calories absolutely need

_____

[§] https://www.bbc.co.uk/sport/get-inspired/47977024

replacing, which is why after a big race you will find me in the queue for TGI Fridays. If it's the London Marathon, you will find me there for two hours before I get a table! After finishing the race and queuing with my vibrating beeper for the appropriate amount of time, I ordered a large rump steak and told the waitress that if they put the chips on (no more carbs!) or gave me the associated side of broccoli (I've just run a marathon, why would I waste my chewing energy on green stuff?) I would sue TGIs!

- Every runner burns enough energy to power a smart phone for one year.

A year! I know marathons are tough but we are really working our arses off, aren't we?

- The combined sweat from all 2018 runners would fill 2,340 bath tubs.

Gross! Only half of that would have come from me if I'd been running that year!

- An average marathon runner loses 1.25cm in height due to spine compression.

Apparently, it does come back the following day after your discs regain fluid. Dave Phillips, MBE is still nearly 6 feet tall despite his 501 marathons, so I don't think we need to worry about shrinkage.

- An average marathon runner takes 50,000 steps in the race.

And unless every one of them are on Strava, it didn't count!

Since becoming a runner, the word 'marathon' has become much more common in my vocabulary but of course it is something I've been vaguely familiar with since I was a child. One primary school teacher, who was absolutely not a runner, explained one day that the marathon we see on the TV was 'invented' in the Ancient Games that took place in Greece circa 776 BC to AD 393.

I've since learned that long-distance running was never included in the Ancient Games but, somewhere along the line, around 490 BC a Greek messenger ran from Marathon to Athens with news of Greek victory over the Persians. The distance was 40 kilometres (24.8 miles for those of you working imperially) and he promptly dropped dead at the finish, after delivering his message. Long-distance running was later introduced to the Olympics and the distance of the 1896 Olympic Marathon was set at 40 kilometres (again, 24-ish miles) to commemorate the life and the run of the Greek Messenger.

But today, every marathon runner knows that 24-ish miles is not a marathon, so when did the extra 1 mile, 385 yards get added? Did someone go the wrong way once and it stuck? Well, actually, rumour has it that at the 1908 games, Queen Alexandra, married to King Edward at the time and residing at Windsor Castle, requested the race begin in the castle grounds so her children could watch from their nursery (getting the kids interested in sport early, I like it!). She wished the finish line to be outside the royal box in the Olympic stadium. The distance was 42.195 kilometres (26.2 miles), which evidently did stick and was formally announced as the Olympic marathon distance in 1921.

I'd be interested to know how that went down with runners at the time! If something changes in a race today, there are immediately 3,700 comments on Facebook declaring it absurd alongside threats of "I'm never gonna do this race again!"

Did the runners of the day take to the streets in protest at the extra distance? Imagine planning to run 24-ish miles and someone comes along and changes it to 26.2 for their own selfish reasons. What would happen today if suddenly the official marathon distance was increased to 27.7 miles? There'd definitely be rioting!

As much as running a marathon feels very commonplace in modern times, I do still think it's something of an elite club.

To me, it's a really impressive distance – 26.2 miles on your own two feet – and I will never be complacent about what a big undertaking it is for a runner, whether new or experienced. I think when you're in a running club, with so many of the people around you taking on marathons without a second thought, it's easy to forget how far, how tough and how incredible running a marathon really is. The prevalence of races increases this forgetfulness and it certainly seems like you could run a marathon anywhere in the world every weekend of the year if you were so inclined. Over the last few years, race companies have even started hosting midweek marathons. Imagine that!

Running a marathon on a Tuesday morning! How commonplace.

"Shall I do this week's big shop today? Nah, I'll just run 26.2 miles."

It feels like the whole world is constantly marathon-ready.

But actually, it's not. By 2018, only 1,298,725 runners had ever finished a marathon. I know that sounds like an awful lot, but in a population of over seven billion it's a drop in the ocean.

Yes, Mr Pedantic Reader out there, I know not every one of those seven billion people would have been able to run a marathon – some would be babies, some would be physically unable and so should be discounted from the stats etc. – but I'm not writing a mathematical account of marathon statistics from around the world. I'm just pointing out that not many of the world's population ever finish a marathon and those who do are pretty special. OK? Jerk!

During the COVID-19 pandemic, running clubs, like everyone, had to close their doors. Races were cancelled, parkrun was halted, running shops had to close and club training sessions ceased. At first, I panicked. I didn't want to lose my connection to the running community and I didn't want that community to dwindle. At the time, I was the social secretary at my running club, along with Jo, and we decided on day one of the lockdown that we had to do whatever we could to keep some semblance of normality for our 200+ runners. Along with other committee members and club mates, we went headfirst into the world of virtual running.

Jo and I commandeered an existing club Facebook group that had been used in the past to organise a running challenge and turned it in a virtual clubhouse, inviting members to share stories and photos from their lockdown lives, whether it was running related or not. We just wanted to keep everyone connected in some way, especially as we had no idea how long the lockdowns would last. At this point runners could take to the outdoors for their daily exercise, albeit separate from any other runners. What previously could be a very social activity suddenly became completely isolated.

We began our virtual running lives with a 'Pass the Vest' challenge. Runners from around the club filmed themselves throwing and catching their iconic red and white running vest whilst engaging in a variety of activities (for example, whilst on a trampoline, whilst dressed as a dinosaur, whilst drinking a glass of wine – all very normal stuff for members of our club) and I edited (not expertly by any means) them into a short video to look like the vest was being passed from runner to runner. It was good fun, but in all honesty I stole the idea from another running club who had done the same thing a few days before! I like to think our runners came up with more novel ways to 'pass the vest' though, particularly the lovely Casey, who was mid-plank when a red and white vest went flying over the top of her and into the hands of the next runner.

To keep our running social lives going we followed this up with a virtual dance off, in which Jo and the energetic Denise tied for top spot – Jo with a very stylised piece to *Proud Mary* and Denise performing a mesmerising rendition of *Lord of The Dance* around her living room. The telly had even been pushed back – these Irish dancers take their craft very seriously.

Our social 'events' continued with virtual karaoke and a lip-sync challenge; again, I seem to recall Jo taking a lead role in most performances. She's quite theatrical! We were treated to a series of videos from our treasurer Norm in which he 'performed' and 'paraded' for us, dancing and singing to a host of catchy tunes. Norm kept us very entertained on a Friday night 'pub' session right up until the Facebook police sent him to Facebook jail for virtual nudity after one of his costumes involved a pair of chaps!

Over the lockdown, our runners took to the group to share news from home. We discussed the ups and downs of solo running and our banana bread highs and lows, all in the name of keeping connected. However, it wasn't just socially that we continued to exist as a running club, but physically too. As much as we could, we changed our training sessions and races to virtual events, starting with our weekly core-strength class, RaceFit, which moved straight to Skype (and, later, Zoom, once we realised that was easier to set up!). I led many of the sessions from the comfort of my living room, along with the rest of the RaceFit team from theirs. In my sessions, runners came to expect lots of wittering, inappropriate comments and me laughing at my own poor jokes. They also came to expect that I would never have my camera in the right position and either my head or feet would always be cut off!

(not)parkrun took off brilliantly and I loved logging my virtual 5k runs each week. I was even able to register my dad and log some of the weekly walks we did, which he really enjoyed. No sooner would we arrive at our finish point and he'd be asking if I'd uploaded it yet and whether we'd been quicker than last week or not. At 83, and set in his ways, joining an in-the-flesh parkrun is out of the question as far as he is concerned, so having a similar experience virtually, without the pressure, was a brilliant addition to our fitness routine in lockdown. He's a very quick walker and walks further than 5k most days but he's worried that at parkrun he'd be last (like so many of us are when we start parkrun, before we know it doesn't matter) or that he'd be frowned upon for walking. We all know this wouldn't be the case and that walking is very much welcomed. In fact, as I write this, tomorrow marks the start of parkwalk month. The whole of October will be dedicated by parkrun UK to encouraging people to come along and walk, whilst soaking up the atmosphere, meeting new people and being active. It shows that the running community welcomes everyone; you don't have to run to be part of it. You can walk, support, volunteer or even just watch and still be part of this great group of people. Some of our older club members who can no longer run still meet up once a week on training night for a catch up and a pint in our clubhouse.

One of the most community-spirited of the lockdown races came in the form of the 'Around the World in 80 Days' challenge, in which five local running clubs competed to be the first whose members could collectively run 24,901 miles – pretty much the distance of running once around the Earth. Every mile counted towards the total, so it really was the most inclusive running event you could hope to take part in. Even if you could only manage a mile or two here and there because of injury, inability or inexperience, it all still counted towards your club's total and that's all that mattered.

The winning club, Kenilworth Runners, completed the distance in an astonishing 37.8 days and there was even talk of them going back around the world for a second attempt! The Massey Runners completed the distance in an impressive 58 days and, along with the other four clubs, and our local running shop Coventry Runner, raised a total of £3,514 in donations and fundraising. The money was presented to University Hospital Coventry and Warwickshire in support of the work they did during the early pandemic. The event prompted a lot of friendly, virtual rivalry and banter between the local clubs and was one of the defining events of lockdown running. Even now, over two years on, you will still see local runners donning their bright green, orange and blue commemorative race vests during training runs.

Another iconic event in local virtual running was the Virtual London Marathon, organised by the brilliant Brenda. If you aren't aware, the London Marathon, like many races, switched to a virtual event in which runners could take on the 26.2 miles in their chosen location, retaining the spirit of the event even in the toughest of times. Brenda rose to the occasion in such a fabulous way, keeping us all running together (but nowhere near each other!). She planned a safe route, organised the setting up and manning of a number of feed and fuel stations and created a buzz and vibe for the day akin to what runners would feel in the regular London-based race. We had a great turnout of runners, spectators and volunteers – all socially distanced but close in spirit. By this point six people could congregate together in outside spaces, so the feed stations were well-manned and supported, fuelling weary runners as they made their way around the streets of Coventry. There were other non-club runners out and about doing their own virtual marathon that day and upon seeing our feed stations, their eyes widened! Of course, they were welcomed with open arms (metaphorically – there was still no touching at this point), especially as our members had stocked the food stations so well that we could have fed the five thousand.

For a number of our club runners, Brenda's Virtual

London Marathon was their first taste of the marathon experience and they have all said they wouldn't change it. It may not have been on the streets of London with tens of thousands of other runners and supporters but it brought us together as a community when we had little other choice. The whole event proved that the running community, and our club in particular, can overcome any hurdle and come out in force to keep running against all odds.

I have to give a further shout out to our Brenda – not only did she organise one of the biggest and most popular events of our club's virtual running period, but she also continues to organise fundraising and social events to support a number of charities, both local and national. Her barn dances are a highlight of our running club social year and her recent breakfast run, in which she and her family fed us sausage batches** and cake following an early morning Sunday run, was one of the nicest running events of the year so far. While the adults earned their sausages on their 5-kilometre or 5-mile runs, Brenda set up a mini fun run for the little ones in attendance, presenting them with a medal and a post-run Fruit Shoot after they navigated a small lap of the nearby field! My 3-year-old niece didn't quite get the memo that she was supposed to run *around* the cones and complete a full lap, instead choosing to cut off half of the little course

---

** To fuel the Great British Bread Debate, you may know a 'batch' as a bread roll, a stottie cake, a cob, a bap or a barm cake!

and make a beeline almost directly for the finish. She still came last! But she enjoyed herself, got her medal and juice and even helped Brenda collect the cones after the race – which is all good practice for when she inevitably succumbs to the lure of the running world. Her mum, uncle and aunty are all runners, so what choice does she have!

In a running club like Massey, where so many runners embody the community spirit I've described above, you won't be surprised to learn that there is room for everyone. Fast, slow, big, small, old, young. There are people who like to run in small groups and those who prefer to run with lots of others. There are runners who never race and runners who race every weekend. There is so much inclusion and support amongst our members that you can be any kind of runner you wish and still be welcomed with open arms.

I myself usually run in one of the three slowest training groups, depending on how I am feeling week by week. Although some might baulk at me singling out some groups as not being as fast as others, I actually have no problem using the word 'slow' – I think it's OK to refer to 'slow runners' or 'slower runners'. It's just an adjective. A descriptive word. I am slower than some runners and faster than others but it doesn't change the fact that we are all runners. I don't expect to be looked down upon by the faster runners and I don't expect the slower runners to judge me as I run past. What I enjoy in Massey Runners is that our members celebrate and support every runner to the same degree, whether they are faster or slower. Recently, one of our fastest club runners came first at parkrun in around 18 minutes. On the same day, one of our runners came almost last, having walked the course. And around 20 of us came somewhere between the two, having either run, Jeffed or walked. Every one of us was congratulated in the same way when we shared our social media posts and photos later that day.

We have a lot of 'Jeffers' these days, which may not be the case in some running clubs, particularly some of the more 'traditional' ones, but in ours, as I think I've made clear, everyone is welcome. A Jeffer, for anyone who hasn't come across the term, is a runner who employs the run/walk technique devised by Olympian Jeff Galloway in the Seventies. It is a race strategy that involves using a very structured pattern of running and walking during a race or training run (e.g. 4-minute run, 1-minute walk), the goal being that the runner can complete longer runs with less toll taken on their body, both physically and mentally. It is a very flexible strategy that many runners adjust to accommodate their own fitness and goals when it comes to endurance running.

I have tried it myself during various runs with some of those in the club who swear by the method and I can see why it works for many. It provides a nice respite from continuous running and allows the legs and lungs to recuperate for a minute. The trouble for me was that I found it hard to concentrate on something so structured and I kept forgetting to walk when I was supposed to (and then I kept forgetting to run again afterwards!). I just like to run without thinking and see what happens. A seasoned runner might take one look at me, eight years into my running 'career', and think "Aw, first timer." I can run, but I can't 'run', if that makes sense… Basically, what I am doing is technically, by the dictionary definition, classed as running but it's not always the kind of running that you might recognise! I just go with the flow and do what works for me in the moment. And that's what so good about running – it can be whatever you want it to be!

When I asked for race report submissions, one of my lovely club mates, Sonia, was quite emphatic about what the experience of virtual running during the pandemic meant to her and how it changed her outlook on running, so of course it's only right that her report features here in the chapter about all of running's best bits! Here she shares a quick note for the reader before telling us about her virtual Chocathon and virtual London Marathon.

Race Report
Sonia's Virtual Races

The biggest point I want to make is that in the initial COVID-19 lockdown and subsequent lockdowns, I really embraced solo running, training and virtual races. My pre-Covid enthusiasm for actual races was such that I took part in two a month on average, as well as satisfying my eager and dedicated parkrun participation and ever-increasing parkrun tourism. In fact, I had such a focus some years ago that I planned to achieve my 300th parkrun on my 60th birthday in November 2021! Yes, I really did calculate it that far in advance!

Pre-Covid, I thought those races and parkruns were so important and despite all the awfulness of the pandemic restrictions, I am just so grateful that I was still able to run solo and then later with my Massey Runners club mates, virtually or in person. Virtual running really did get me through those very strange times.

Sonia

Without a ballot place for the London Marathon, my friend Mylénè and I signed up for the Tissington Trail Marathon, scheduled for 26th April 2020, the same day as London Marathon.

Training started in the New Year and included a half marathon and a 20-miler as part of the preparation. At this point, we were hearing the first reports of COVID-19 reaching the UK. By 15th March, when several of my Massey Runner club mates turned up alongside me for the Oundle 20 in Northamptonshire, we all feared it would be our last 'real' race for a while. We were not wrong.

Very quickly, my next races – two half marathons and a 10k – were either postponed or cancelled altogether. Still, I hung onto the fact that I had another 10k and 10-miler booked for Autumn 2020, and these fitted quite well with the now rescheduled date of 22nd November for the Tissington Trail Marathon.

In the early lockdown weeks I was just grateful that I was allowed to run at all – and then overjoyed when it was announced we could meet up with our running buddies in small bubbles. Also, by this point the virtual race world had opened up and I had the Massey Runners Remote Relays, the Kenilworth Grand Prix, the Warwickshire Road Race League and many other charity virtual races to give my training the focus it needed, and to have something to look forward to.

Marathon training started again in August with weekly long slow runs, usually on Fridays. When Brenda organised a virtual London Marathon event in October it was win-win, because I could support my running friend Amanda, who would be taking part along with various other club mates, whilst doing a 16-mile long slow run myself. The joys of that Sunday were short-lived because a few days later the Tissington Trail Marathon was postponed again, this time until 2021. Despite all the COVID-19 measures the organisers had put in place, the landowners would no longer allow the race to go ahead.

I did find some replacement marathon options for November and opted for the Saxons, Vikings and Normans Northampton Chocathon. My choice was based on the date, its proximity to my home city, a naive belief that it wouldn't be cancelled and the lure of lots of chocolate goodies over a 5-ish lap course!

Oh, how wrong I was. Instead, lockdown number two came along. With training completed and faced with yet another marathon postponed until 2021, I decided to take the virtual Chocathon option that the organisers offered.

The great thing about this was the opportunity not only to decide my own race date and start time, but to choose my own route. This meant plotting several laps, heading out from and returning to my car on my friends Angela and Dave's drive so I could refuel, while making each lap shorter than the last to give myself some sort of psychological edge. Added to that, I included local routes that I really enjoy running.

Although I had none of the usual cheering and water stations you get along the route at real races, at least I didn't have pre-race nerves – and no waiting around for my wave start. Instead, I had the incredible support of Massey Runners tracking my progress on iPhones and co-ordinating their arrival so they could start the next lap with me. There were even strategic race photographers (thank you, Janette and Andy), and Angela handed out my chocolate goody bags as a little thank you to my lap-running buddies.

Angela, Dave, Mylénè, Amanda, Debbie, Sheila, Janette and Andy – you all gave amazing support before, during and after the race. You helped the miles fly by and showed just how Massey Runners turn up trumps. I really cannot thank you all enough.

I signed up for an actual race as soon as they were back on, but I now also think virtual races are just as much fun, if not more so. So, if there are any runners looking for support for their virtual races, please shout out because I am sure you will find willing volunteers. Especially me!

Chapter Eight
...The Bad and The Ugly

Before we get into this chapter, I want it known that I was having a mental block the day I started writing it and so, for the first time, I utilised a technique I learned called 'free writing'.

Free writing involves typing as fast as is reasonably possible, with no breaks or breathers, for a self-assigned amount of time – I chose 10 minutes. The main rule is that you cannot use the backspace or delete key and if you hit a wall you simply have to type random words or letters just to keep going. Basically, whatever you do, don't stop typing until the time is up.

My 10 minutes began with the utterly elegant and articulate sentence: "Urgh how embarrassing can race photos be. Why are mine always of me sticking out my tongue, why is my mouth always open, why do my legs always look like corned beef hmm hmmm errr what shall I write now kggkdgjvnv ldsljf oh sod this."

What I wanted to express was that running photographs, even the ones taken by the official photographer, are usually unflattering. Well, mine are at least; you may have gotten away with a few good ones yourself. For me, it always looks like I am sinking into the ground, which, in turn, is forcing all my leg fat to gather up around my thighs. On a cold day especially, my legs look as if they're made of corned beef and that doesn't come across well in race photographs (or in real life).

The ideal, but elusive, race photo is of course the one with 'flying feet', where you have achieved such speed and velocity in your run that you no longer need one foot on the ground for balance and stability. You are basically gliding through the air in sure and certain hope of a podium finish. Or at least a PB. I don't recall having a 'flying feet' photograph but I do have one where I only look mildly drunk and disorderly, so that's good. That one's in a frame on my sideboard.

The latest craze in mid-race posing for the camera comes in the form of 'the jump'. If you are not familiar with this, the runner about to be photographed takes an enormous leap into the air with both feet very much off the ground, kicks their heels up and offers a double thumbs up or similar to the photographer. It's quite an impressive feat and makes for an excellent race photo; if you're not going to look good running, look good leaping instead. I am never going to try 'the jump' – it would be foolish of me even to consider it when I trip over imaginary sticks and slip off every kerb I encounter on a run. My attempt would no doubt be redubbed 'the heap' as I lie, immortalised in a photo, in a pile on the ground, legs and arms everywhere, feet no longer facing the direction in which nature intended.

A lot of runners throw their arms up in the air in a

victorious fashion when approaching the race photographer. I thought this might be something far more achievable for me than 'the jump' or anything quite so adventurous, so I've been giving it a go over a few different races. What I've found is that whilst everybody else looks like they are jubilantly celebrating a win, I look like I am carrying an invisible box over my head – my arms just don't look right. There's too much bend at the elbows, like I am bracing for a heavy weight. I am going to run an Instagram competition shortly to see who can photoshop the most ridiculous items into my hands. The winner will probably get a signed copy of this book!

In my most absurd race photograph you will find me half in, half out of the shot (that's really on the photographer, not me) with one arm half in the air, the other reaching out and around to the side like I am hugging the invisible man (OK, the photographer can't do much about that) and my tongue hanging out of the side of my mouth like a sleeping puppy. I appear to be moving sideways rather than forward. I should be mortified by it but I choose to embrace it and, through regular sharing of it on my Instagram, I have come to realise why all my running photos are so bad.

It's my face.

And my body.

I can't put the blame on the photographers!

Occasionally, it is not the cameras pointing at you that cause the most embarrassment but the ones you pass mid-run that are pointing at others. This is a fairly niche running experience, so if you are not quite sure what I am referring to, don't worry; I will explain.

If you are out running in the Cotswolds, say around leg four of the Hilly 100 route, you will find yourself immersed in picturesque countryside and quaint village life. You will also find yourself facing what is described by many as the longest hill in the world. I'm not sure if it really is the longest hill in the world but the severity of a hill – or a mound of opportunity, as my amazing friend Kelli calls them – is subjective.

And it was Kelli who stumbled across the alternative awkward camera experience – the shooting of an 'adult' movie whilst she was completing leg four of the race. As Kelli explains, she was making her way up "that blimmin' longest hill" when three people came into view across the glorious vista. Two ladies dressed in cat ears, jackets and boots (nothing else?) were standing close to where a rotund bearded gentleman was setting up a video camera. Of course, it may not have been an adult movie but to everyone who passed them during the race that day, it appeared to be the case. If it barks like a dog and all that… Plus how many everyday scenarios involve the wearing of cat ears and take place in the woods in front of a video camera?

Kelli told me she was unsure what to do as she passed, so she simply gave the cast a polite, respectful nod. My dear Kelli, a polite nod is what you do when passing fellow runners, not porn stars (although I suppose they could be runners too). Our fabulous friend Tiffanie, who ran the same leg of the race but for another team, confirmed she just stared at them as she passed. There was no knowing head nod in acknowledgement from Tiff. I think she made the right call; Kelli's acknowledgement could have been mistaken by the cast members for a knowing nod of approval and they may have beckoned her over!

Recently, my brother-in-law Simon asked how the book was coming along and we got talking about running for quite some time. At this point in his life, particularly as he is married to Jo, he should know better than to bring up running with a runner but he is clearly a glutton for punishment.

At some point in our lengthy conversation, in which I probably did most of the talking, Simon managed to squeeze in an anecdote about a party he once attended. While there he struck up a conversation with someone he knew to be a runner. Not knowing a great deal about running at that point, but with good intentions, he decided to go out on a limb and ask: "So, I bet you've done one of those muddy runs?"

Muddy runs, if you don't know, tend to be the charitable 5km and 10km races that many women, men and children take part in, usually for fun, fitness and to raise money for charity. They are great fun, a significant challenge for many and raise vital funds and awareness. What Simon hadn't realised was that the runner he was talking to was in fact a running snob who would take offence to the words 'muddy' and 'run' being spoken in their vicinity. Simon promptly had his head cleanly bitten off for daring to suggest a runner of this calibre would participate in something as banal as a 'fun run'.

Unfortunately, as great as running is, it can attract the occasional running snob and/or nob. Of course, I don't mind anyone taking pride in whatever aspect of running they feel strongly about or are good at, be it pace, distance, frequency and so on. I just don't like it when runners look down on others because they are achieving or striving towards different things.

The pace snob is a runner who doesn't consider anything below their pace to be 'running'. If you are slower than them, you are beneath them on their perceived scale of runner-ness! You'll know you've encountered one because they try to hide their contempt for you by pretending to encourage you to improve your pace, but they won't ever fully engage with you until you reach their 'gold standard' running pace.

Don't try and tell them you 'ran' a 5k in 35 minutes, or you'll be met with: "Oh, you *jogged* a 5k, that's nice." They never ask, "Did you enjoy that?" or "How was your race?" The only conversation starter they can muster up is "How fast did you do it?" When they ask me that, they have usually walked away from me before I even finish sharing the details.

The distance snob is much like the pace snob. They have a perceived notion of how far a 'real runner' can travel and if you fall below this, you are fair game to be trampled over next time they lap you in a race. They usually only ask you how your race went in the hope that it will elicit a response of "And yours?" so they can brag about their superior mileage.

The kit snob is the one who scoffs at your supermarket own brand active wear and spits on your shoes as they race past you in their carbon-soled Zoomieflys. (If that's a real brand, I apologise!) If these snobs knew how old my favourite sports bra is, they might vomit! When it comes to kit, for the average runner money doesn't buy you many gains. Sometimes I wear a pair of £59.99 twin-layer shorts but I have to stop every four minutes to 'retrieve' them from somewhere quite private, and other times I wear a pair of £9.99 twin-layer shorts I've had since 2015 that haven't ridden up even once.

The "I don't train" snob is always quite vocal about never needing to train and their God-given ability to just crack out miles at the drop of a hat. They are almost an inverted snob with their opinion that anyone who works towards their goal is a 'sell-out', contributing to the gentrification of running. Their worst nightmare would be to be 'just like the rest of us' meagre mortal runners.

The "I'm a natural" snob is possibly the worst, although they can't really help it, so I don't have too much contempt for them. They are naturally gifted in all aspects of running. They are fast, can run for miles and their kit always looks pristine. Their sweat smells of Zoflora Country Garden. They only engage with others of their kind but you can spot them by the hordes of adoring fans lying at their feet after a race!

The "I was nearly a doctor" snob has a degree in medicine from the University of Rainbows and Unicorns and had planned to become a doctor but had a tummy ache the day they were supposed to apply. They still like to impart medical advice, however, specialising in "It's not good news" outcomes with all the bedside manner of a binbag. My favourite quote of theirs is: "I had that; you'll never run properly again." (All I had was a splinter from walking barefoot on the decking!) This particular snob doesn't understand the difference between sharing their own experience in case someone else might benefit and telling someone exactly what to do and how to do it. I've had a lot of injuries myself (I've got a dodgy left side!) and I do get asked for advice, or sometimes it comes up naturally, and I'm always careful to add, "But that's just me, you might be different." It's the perfect catch-all!

The foodie snob shares the same photo of their protein shake and energy ball breakfast every morning alongside the screenshot of their Strava. They never eat cake, and I personally don't think you can trust any runner who doesn't eat cake! Their post-run 'treat' is usually a beetroot smoothie made with Italian ass's milk and a side of spinach.

The anti-fun snob will not give you the time of day

if you try to tell them about your colour run, the fun run you did with your mum or that obstacle course you did with the girls from work. They are not interested unless it was two back-to-back Tough Mudders in the Sahara Desert, at night, and you were blindfolded. Which they already did last year while suffering a broken leg.

If you dare to do a race in fancy dress, they will deny all knowledge of your existence and erase every trace of you from their life. If you see them, they will look through you. If you talk about your 'novelty' race near them, they will sarcastically ask those around, "Did you hear something?"

So the big question now is: which running snob am I? Which one are you?

OK, it would be nice to think I don't display any of these traits as a runner (and neither do you), but I'm only human and I know I occasionally get caught up with aspects of running that are just not important to everyone. I actually think I have the potential to be any or all of the running snobs at any given time, depending on my own personal situation, emotions, hormones or mental wellbeing. I'm certainly not perfect; I'm part of a WhatsApp group called Running Gossip Girls, where we rant and rave about the runners who have wronged us and damn them to hell for all eternity.

If you're pretending to act shocked, calm down!

Everyone has a dark side – even you, probably –

and being a bitch can be quite cathartic if it's just in your head and doesn't hurt anyone else physically, mentally, emotionally, or otherwise. I hold my hands up and confess that I have looked at a person's Strava and in my bad mood (at the time) muttered to myself, "Was it even worth going out?" or "LOL she thinks that's a hill!" Of course, I genuinely don't believe those things and would never say them to anyone directly (not because I'm two-faced, but because I believe that not everything you think needs to be said, especially when it benefits no one and is only a fleeting thought!) but we do all have the capacity to be a little judgemental or competitive. It's like we have our own personal running devil sitting on our shoulder. Most of us hide it well and would never use it in a way that makes someone else feel bad; it's often just an internal voice that you can't control because you're otherwise engaged in a bad mood or difficult situation. Or, if you're like me, just hungry. Or tired. Or cold.

If you have never had a bad thought about another runner, you are to be commended. If you're more like me, however, you will have a list of runners (not an actual written-down list; that would be sociopathic) who you don't really gel with and who, in return, quite dislike you. But when you see each other in a race you will cheer, chat and support each other like decent human beings before going back to your trashy WhatsApp group to act like an inverted snob and criticise their £100 designer leggings that you secretly wish you had!

I dread to think how many times I've been the subject of someone's WhatsApp group chat:

"OMG, did you see Jenna vomiting on the finish line? What a tramp!"

"Did you see her arse in those cheap leggings?"

If Santa Claus keeps a record of these runners on his naughty list, alongside the snobs you might also see the names of the rule-breakers. These are the runners who live life on the edge, not afraid to get caught for taking a risk and doing what they like. They are the runners who wear headphones when it's strictly prohibited (shock horror!), or the runners who give away their race place to someone else even though the terms and conditions forbid it (I am appalled!).

If you read the terms of any race, you'll almost always see that there are no transfers allowed, or at least no 'rogue' transfers where you just swap numbers. The reason behind this is quite simply safety. The organisers need to know exactly who is participating in their event should something untoward occur, like an accident. Some races operate a legitimate transfer scheme but in most, an entry is non-transferable. This means that if something crops up meaning you can't race, you have two choices – abide by the 'law' and forego the entry, or live dangerously and give the place away. I have always stayed on the right side of the law and it's meant that I've pulled out of many races, losing my entry fee and missing out on a medal. There was that one time, however, when I was an accomplice to my brilliant friend Lisa and her rule-breaking ways.

When Lisa signed up for A. N. Other race (I'm not going to include the actual race name in case the organisers read this and ban us both from running in their future events!), she did so in good faith, planning to train hard and attempt a PB. As it often does, life got in the way and shortly before race day she decided it was best to forego the race and talked me into taking her place in an 'off book' transfer i.e. she gave me her bib number and I gave her 10 quid. I do generally like to do things by the book and honestly (as far as I can remember!), this was the one and only time I took someone else's number, except where legitimate transfers were offered.

As Lisa handed me the race bib, I noticed it was very jazzy. Too jazzy, maybe? It was very glossy, with a yellow background and black and white stripes. I figured a lot of money went into this race's consumables. She also handed me the lucky dollar. I had previously given her a dollar bill I won in Las Vegas and we arbitrarily decided it was lucky – even though it never showed any signs of bringing either of us good or back luck in a race! (NB The dollar bill is entirely irrelevant to this story but, as mentioned earlier, I have over 200 pages to fill and using lots of extra words that are entirely unnecessary is how I intend to fill those when the actual running content runs out!)

On race day, I made my way to the start line. It's a big race, thousands of runners, and I started to notice the rainbow of colours on their race bibs... pink, green, blue, orange, white... not many stripy ones like mine (well, Lisa's). Where were all the other stripy ones?

As I looked for the entrance to my start corral, which would be indicated by a sign of the same colour, I started to notice fewer and fewer runners who looked like me and more and more Beautiful People. (I mentioned the Beautiful People, didn't I? Tall, leggy, svelte, glossy hair, run like the wind!) As I walked the length of the corrals, the shorts were getting shorter, runners were getting taller (maybe that's why the shorts were getting shorter?), and everyone was looking much slenderer than me; they actually had calf muscles. I also noticed that no one in these particular corrals was taking selfies like I usually do pre-race, and instead seemed to be partaking in some form of dynamic stretching.

I eventually found the entrance to my start corral, which was marked by a large yellow, black and white stripy sign matching my race bib and was emblazoned with the words 'Fast Club Runners'. It turns out Lisa had wildly overestimated her time – she claims it was a mistake with a missing zero on her application, but I wouldn't put it past her that she'd done it on purpose so she could run, however briefly, amongst the tanned and toned Beautiful People. She is a bit of a wild one!

As I stood amongst them, mostly looking up, I

remembered I could drop back a corral and run with others who were perhaps more closely matched to my own ability. Unfortunately, I was too penned in by The Beautiful People and the start time was rapidly approaching. I didn't think I'd have time to get out of the corral and wander back to a later one, so I stood there, short and awkward.

I rubbed my calf a little and made 'ouch' noises so maybe they'd think I was normally a Fast Club Runner but had injured myself today. To be fair, I did have a club vest on, so that ticked the 'club' box. I was just missing the 'fast' part.

Seconds after the start klaxon sounded for our wave ('our' wave – again, I'm talking like I belonged there!), there wasn't a single Fast Club Runner in sight. They had left me for dust, quite as I had expected. Worse still, it wasn't long before the front of the subsequent wave, presumably the 'Less Fast but Still Fast Enough Club Runners', caught me from behind.

I did have a good run though – for me, that is, not for a Fast Club Runner. I was actually only a minute off my race PB for that distance – which, when you consider that this was the race when I stopped to use the potentially dodgy industrial estate portaloo, I don't think is too shabby.

And then there's Stuart, the second rule breaker in this household.

Three weeks before his second attempt at Ironman

Vichy, Stuart was offered a place in a local triathlon by a friend of his, Paul, who was no longer able to race. There were absolutely no transfers allowed in this race; however, this didn't stop Stuart gladly accepting the offer and 'illegally' taking over Paul's race place! He felt it would be a nice tester for the forthcoming big event and that he would just take it gently and enjoy it. I went along on the day to offer my services as a marshal on the course. I thought it might balance out the race-day Karmic debt from Stuart's blatant disregard for the transfer rules.

I watched him set off on his swim and then collected my hi-vis and volunteer's packed lunch and walked a few miles out to where I would be marshalling for the day. I spent the next few hours cheering on runners, lap after lap, eventually seeing some of them for the third time as they headed into their final lap before finishing. It took me a while but eventually it dawned on me that I hadn't yet seen Stuart. Being a multi-lap course and Stuart being a fairly OK triathlete, I figured it was a bit odd, but I'm not brilliant on calculating timings so I didn't give it too much thought.

Plus I was too busy cheering on the runners, including my friend Sam to whom I made a mildly offensive comment, the kind that only a real friend can make. Sam didn't laugh at all and I was worried I had finally found the line between banter and offence. It was only when I saw Sam a few minutes later that I realised the former Sam was not my Sam! I had cheered and been borderline obscene to a very random, confused stranger. Lesson learnt: always wait until someone is close enough that you can read their name on their vest before you shout obscenities.

Another hour of cheering passed. I'd been delivered my first snack pack by the race organisers and was eagerly awaiting the volunteer burger drop off and the volunteer ice cream delivery when, out in the distance, I spotted a race official barrelling towards me, shouting: "Are you Jenna?"

Bizarrely, that's a difficult question to answer when a stranger says your name.

"Am I Jenna?"

"Why does this stranger know my name?"

"Does he have my burger?"

He finally reached me, sweaty and panting, and, through spluttered speech, told me: "Everything's OK but there's been an accident and Paul's fallen off his bike."

"Do I know a Paul?" I wondered. Well, yes I do, but not in this race, and certainly not a Paul that I am so closely connected to that a race official would feel the need to run 2 miles into the countryside just to tell me there'd been an accident.

Then I realised. Stuart had taken Paul's bib number.

Paul = Stuart. Stuart = Paul.

The officials and first aiders were clearly under the impression he was called Paul, based on the race number emblazoned all over his bike, helmet, arms and legs, and were frantically trying to treat a man who evidently was so hurt he no longer knew his own name!

The moral of this story? Don't swap bib numbers unofficially or you might make more work for the poor paramedics trying to help you out who can't even get a straight answer when they ask you your name. Plus, think of the family. Luckily, Stuart (AKA Paul) was lucid enough that when the officials were talking about phoning his wife he could send them out onto the course to find me instead of calling Paul's unsuspecting actual wife, telling her he'd been in an accident.

Having said that, transferring a race place legitimately is not always without danger. You might end up having the same experience I did and witness a running clubmate in a way-too-short, threadbare bathrobe! (Clearly not as risky as what Stuart did but still traumatic)

It was a few weeks before the Two Castles race. If you are not familiar with this race, you start at one castle (Warwick) and run to another castle (Kenilworth) for a total of 10k.

I had not been lucky enough to get a place in the ballot but saw on Facebook that one of The Beautiful People was giving away their place. This race allows transfers up until a certain date, so it would all be totally legitimate. I pinged off a quick message to snap up the place but I was too late. It had already gone to another runner; however, The Beautiful Person mentioned someone else they had heard of who was giving up a place. The place was being offered by one of our club's Lifetime Members – a Lifetime Member, for your information, has at least 15 years' consecutive membership and has contributed widely to the success of the club. It's something I aspire to achieve.

This particular member has always called me Rachel to this day. I have never corrected him, so it's 50/50 my fault too. I think he knows who I am because he asks the right questions when I bump into him, just always under the name Rachel. It's a nice name though, so I'm fine with it.

I reached out to the Lifetimer who confirmed the place was mine; he'd done the transfer online and just needed me to pop around with the £15 fee and to collect the bib number. I went later that day; I was really keen to do this race, so I wanted to get hold of the bib straight away.

When he opened his front door, I found myself greeted by a very cheery man dressed in a short – very short – threadbare robe. "Hi Rachel, come in," he offered.

I had only planned to stand at the door but I'm polite, so I stepped into the dining room. From the living room, I heard his wife shout: "Jenna does not need to see you in your little robe!"

Lifetimer looked down, realised he was nearly nude, tightened his robe and said: "Sorry, Rachel…" (am I in an episode of *Only Fools and Horses* here?) then carried on chit chatting to me politely for an extraordinary lengthy amount of time. As time went on the robe reopened and was closed numerous times, while I continued to politely take part in the conversation whilst maintaining a strong, solid glare out of the window to my right side.

"Yep."

"Hmm."

"Sure."

I kept briefly responding, politely nodding but never making eye contact or fully engaging in the conversation. He must've thought I had a cricked neck!

If I'd been interested in creating maximum awkwardness, this really should have been the time I finally corrected him on the name discrepancy. "Sorry, but once again, can you please just cover up your penis... Oh, and by the way, it's Jenna."

Quick and painless. Just massively awkward.

Next time I will forget running the race and just go watch instead!

As well as the rule breakers and the running snobs, there is a third type of runner that provides good content for an amateur writer who needs to hit a 70,000+ word count with a deadline approaching: runners who offer totally unsolicited advice, particularly when that advice is neither correct nor relevant.

I recently saw a running meme on Instagram that

said: "Opinions are like penises. Just because you have one and you think it's great doesn't mean you should share it in public when no one asked."

It's possible that sharing running advice has become the equivalent of sending a dick pic without prior permission. Thankfully, I've never received a dick pic (please don't see that as a challenge, dear reader) but I have had lots of unsolicited running advice over the years. Of course, some of it has been great and has helped me overcome various hurdles. Like Dave telling me to dress for mile 2, or Paul advising me to visualise the finish line when I'm struggling.

Unfortunately, however, lots of it has been useless or, in some cases, quite harmful.

There is one particular member of my running community who pokes me in the ribs every time they see me and provides these words of caution: "You're running too much; you've lost too much weight."

I know it seems unlikely when I've previously explained how great it is to be part of a running club but, as we established, it isn't always a perfect running world.

The rib-poker doesn't know me very well. Those who do know me well would never accuse me of running too much! Just this week I was corrected by Stuart about the number of times per week I've been running lately. I've been proudly telling people that I am back to running three times per week after my injuries, but Stuart politely and quietly pointed out that training on a Wednesday and parkrun on a Saturday does not equate to three days.

Somehow, at 37 years old, I miscalculated the number of days in a week.

If anything, I've been running less than ever, so I don't know why Pokey Joe (disclaimer, they are not called Joe) keeps digging me in the ribs and telling me I should go to the doctor's to get checked out. Combined with the pandemic and the comfort eating that went with it, I most certainly have not lost weight through running. But, nonetheless, this person likes to poke me in the ribs with a disgusted scoff and tell me I "look like a stick."

I'm not sure I understand the interaction. Do they genuinely think I've lost weight and they're concerned? If so, there are politer ways to put it. Maybe they are due a trip to Specsavers or they have sweat in their eyes from running. I don't want to get too heavy here, as that's not the theme of this book, but my guess is that they associate running with being skinny and perhaps aren't achieving that themselves with their own running. Who knows really? I try not to let it bother me. I just get straight onto my Gossip Girls WhatsApp group and rant, "You won't believe what they've said now!" with the appropriate number of angry face emojis (three tends to be about right!) and I usually end up feeling better pretty quickly.

Whilst this chapter, on the whole, has been about some of the less positive aspects of running, I didn't want to end it that way. Worried that we'd all be feeling a bit blah at this point, I've chosen a positive, upbeat race report from my clubmate Paul. Paul tells us about his great experience at the Great North Run, a race that I was expecting to love but actually felt quite underwhelmed by. I think I was suffering emotionally after putting all my energy into a big race the weekend before. I didn't hate it; it just felt hard and, a few years down the line, I don't have any great recollections from the day other than that I got straight into the car and left South Shields after the race, rather than heading to the pub with my friends, which is not like me. After reading Paul's race report, I definitely think I need to go back and try it again.

Race Report
Paul's Great North Run

I'd signed up for the Leamington Spa Half Marathon 2020, because I wanted a challenge and I thought I'd raise some money while I was at it. My son is autistic, so the National Autistic Society was my charity of choice. Training was slow but I made progress. The winter of 2019 was great and I'd certainly caught the running bug. And then the world stopped.

I'd already raised some money by this point when it was announced that the event wasn't taking place, so I signed up for the Coventry Half Marathon instead. Then that was postponed…

Forward to 2021 and things seemed somewhat better, and there was still money in my Go Fund Me account. I looked through the National Autistic Society website and saw the Great North Run. It was huge, the biggest half marathon in the world. For my first one, I thought, *Go big or go home!*

I'd trained as much as I could and the time came to drive to Newcastle on the Saturday morning. A long drive with a stop to walk around Leeds, and before I knew it, I could see the Angel of The North on my right as I headed into Newcastle. I'd booked myself into Newcastle Airport Travelodge and arrived early evening. Forward planning is not my strong point and I hadn't considered how far it was to the start of the race, how I was going to get there, or what I was going to do with my car, as I needed to leave it way beyond check-out time. A quick message to a Twitter friend who lives in Newcastle and I had all the information I needed. The chap on the hotel desk said that a few people were leaving their cars for the race and I was welcome to do so too. With all that sorted, it was a carb-loaded carvery at the Toby next door, a bath, and an early night.

Pete (my Twitter friend) had given me some pretty amazing information for the following morning. A short walk to the Metro and I was headed into the city centre with a lot of like-minded folks. You could feel the atmosphere building throughout. Everything was well signposted, and everything seemed… cleaner. Electric scooters weren't just racked as they should be but had helmets too. Crazy!

The meeting point was on the Town Moor, so off I went. I could see the start point as I crossed the bridge, with all the runners in earlier waves already starting off. As I got to the main field, you could hear commentary on who was about to win the elite race. There was a lot of hanging around and not much to do. I had a look around the charity village but nervous energy made me want to keep moving. I finally decided to sit down with a coffee and a Mars Bar as the Red Arrows flew over for the first time. An iconic sight at this great event and if you blinked, you would miss it.

Due to the restrictions that were put in place to keep people safe, the waves of runners were hugely staggered. I could see people on the other side of the moor who were walking across with their finishers' medals and goody bags and I hadn't even got down to the start point yet! A lot of runners who were in far better shape than me were coming across, some limping, some being helped. This didn't fill me with confidence! But, soon enough, my wave was called and we made our way up the hill.

There were a few thousand in my wave. While we were waiting, there was a compere keeping us entertained. He was explaining why the event had had to be changed. The irony of him explaining how they were doing what they could to assist with social distancing while we were all strangers standing almost shoulder to shoulder wasn't lost! There was a charity clothes drop off for anything you didn't want to take with you, so I took off the fleece that was keeping me warm and dropped it on the pile. It was a great thing knowing that all the clothes would be donated. It was also a final chance to grab some water.

I walked up the hill, watching where I put my feet on the uneven ground – a wrong step now would spell disaster when I was so close. The nerves were really kicking in as I went through the barrier on to the main road. I'd made a playlist to keep me entertained on the way round but there was no phone signal as I began the walk to the start point. This was probably a good thing as there were literally thousands of people lining the roads and bridges cheering you on. I started my watch and off I went.

After the first mile, I saw a large group of runners

on the opposite side who were all going at quite a pace. At that point, I didn't realise that they were on mile 11 on their way back in! I soon settled into my run and listened to the crowd. Crossing the Tyne Bridge for the first time was an amazing experience. Mile 3 became 4 became 5. I had been running steadily uphill for a while and I was glad to reach the turnaround point just before the 10k mark – as what goes up must come down! Even away from the centre into Gateshead, people were still out in force cheering you on. There was so much to keep you distracted along the route.

What big run would be complete without fancy dress? I ran with dinosaurs, three pandas and countless superheroes. I saw the outfit of the day when I hit mile 8. The guy wearing it was clearly a gym lover, muscles everywhere. Probably not much cardio. He looked like he was struggling a little, and on the back of his bright pink top was printed "If you can read this, you didn't train either!"

As I said, what goes up must come down, but unfortunately on this route, the opposite was also true. Due to the course change, the out-and-back route meant the downhills I'd enjoyed at the start had to be run back up. Mile 9 and I was done in. I didn't think I could carry on. Everything hurt. The road turned a corner and the hill got steeper. Another turn and another steep incline and we were on the flyover heading back into the centre of Newcastle.

An old customer of mine who also ran had spoken

to me previously about his half marathons. He gave me a great piece of advice. He told me to get to 10 miles and if I got that far, I'd done it. It was now just a long run with a parkrun on the end, and I knew I could do a parkrun! The crowds were still in force as we made our way back across the Tyne Bridge, telling us that we were nearly there. I certainly needed all the power-up high-fives the crowd were giving out.

And then it was there. At the end of what seemed like the longest road in the world, I could see the finish line in the distance. My legs wanted to stop. My brain wanted to stop. My ego wanted the finish video to have me actually running across the line! So I did. Two hours, 38 minutes and 10 seconds after starting, I'd done my first half marathon. I'd aimed for 2 hours 30 but I was still pleased. I crossed the finish line, stopped my watch, and cried. The emotion got the better of me. I picked up my medal, had my photo taken and took a well-deserved rest.

The walk back to the Metro was tough. There was nothing left in the tank. The path was a long downhill and I could already tell that stairs for the next couple of days would not be my friend. I got back to my car and made the long journey home, stopping off to eat whatever junk food I could find because I'd earned it.

If anyone is thinking of doing the Great North Run, just go for it – whether it's a ballot place or a charity one. Book your hotel early so you can get one close but bear in mind that they can be super expensive for the weekend. The Metro links are great and I can't say enough good things about the Geordies. They're such a warm, welcoming group of people and they help to make the Great North Run what it is.

Chapter Nine
The Injury Bench

In the years I've been running, I've noticed there are two main ways that runners handle being injured. You may be the kind of runner who:

- won't believe, accept or acknowledge that you have even the slightest injury and you continue to run against all advice, or
- believes every little ache or pain marks the end of your running career

I do wonder if the second kind just like to give themselves the opportunity to make a big comeback on a regular basis. Everyone loves a good comeback story! I've had many of my own, although some were more successful than others. Following my latest injury, I'm back to running but I don't feel I've quite made a comeback. There's been nothing triumphant about my return to running this time; I'm just plodding along.

Actually, thinking about my own approach to injuries, let's make that three ways we handle being on the injury bench. You may also be the third kind of runner who:

- bends the truth about the extent of your injuries depending on how it suits you at the time

Yes. That last one is very much my approach.

At any given time, I may be entertaining either of the following split personalities:

Me, excited for a certain race: "Oh, I'm pretty sure that large bone sticking out of my leg will make its way back in by Sunday. What's it called, the femur? Well, I'll just get through this race and then call the doctor Monday if it hasn't sorted itself out."

Also me, tired and grumpy (and probably hungry), regretting signing up for the race in the first place: "Ahhh I grazed my leg on a bush during my trail run. It's agony! I'm going to be sensible and have three months off running. But don't worry, friends, I will be back!" *Dramatically fans face with hand to fight back tears.*

Actually, a lot of the time we do forget that running hurts. It causes trauma to the soft tissues in our bodies and its repetitive nature is often responsible for various injuries. Perhaps we all need to wise up to these facts when it comes to our approach to running injuries. We have to balance an awareness that our bodies are capable of getting broken and they need time to heal but also acknowledge that we can't freak out about every ache and pain.

Some of them are to be expected and not necessarily detrimental, for example DOMS – or delayed onset muscle soreness, to give it its full name – which is the inflammation of tissue that can occur following certain forms of exercise and is very commonly experienced in the aftermath of a run. I'm always amazed by how many runners have never heard of DOMS, considering it often explains the aches and pains felt a few days after running. Instead of gently helping their body to repair with ice, light stretching, a short rest and massage, they immediately put themselves firmly on that sad lonely injury bench.

Of course, there are also those of us who ignore DOMS entirely … Stuart … and just keep piling on the pain by running repeatedly and never giving our tissues time to repair in between. If we would only allow ourselves to rest it could actually lead to increased strength and less chance of injury, prolonging our running career. But many of us runners are inclined towards instant gratification and would rather have bragging rights now about all the running we do than secure our longevity in the sport.

As runners, we could perhaps educate ourselves better – and I include myself in that, wholeheartedly. I have rarely done the 'right thing' for my body as a runner and I imagine I will continue on the same path until the point where all I do is moan about my failing runner's body and how it isn't fair!

Not that I would wish a running injury on anyone, of course I wouldn't, but you'll often hear me grumbling mildly, with all due respect, about those runners who never get injured. Particularly those who do all the 'wrong' things. Jo can run in years-old trainers that are hanging on by a thread and barely get so much as a sore toe. The second my trainers show even the slightest wear and tear, I will be pulling muscles I didn't know I had. Flippancy aside, the only time I have ever heard Jo complain of a running injury was the time she actually did have a slightly sore toe just before parkrun. By mile 1, she had run it off and she's never mentioned it again. Bitch.

My first injury was Achilles tendinopathy and/or Achilles tendonitis. I hear it called different things by different sports therapists and I don't think anyone has ever explained the difference between the two. If you are interested in the difference, if there is any, you'll have to Google it! I suspect it's probably the same condition on the whole, but don't quote me. In fact, I should have said this much earlier but don't quote me on anything in this book please, as it is mostly crap.

As I mentioned earlier, the injury came a month and a half into my new-found hobby of running when I increased my mileage so rapidly, in poor shoes, and without any guidance or input from an expert. I didn't ask any experts for guidance so that's my fault, but at the same time, all I kept hearing was "You're amazing, you're doing so well!"

I'm not complaining. I'm guilty of this myself. We all want to be the motivation and inspiration behind someone else's running – but we tend to forget that we owe it to them to be more realistic. No one wants to be the running bore explaining to an excited new runner about that time you had to have your legs surgically reattached after a race. But you could be saving them from learning the hard way about leg reattachment. (Don't panic, new runners, I'm being hyperbolic to make my point. I don't know of any runner who had their legs fall off after a race.)

The Achilles tendinopathitisism (or whatever it's called) caught me out of the blue. I had run on the Saturday and by Tuesday I didn't even have any sign of DOMS and was preparing for a holiday to America in two days' time. I was walking around the town centre picking up last minute essentials (PG Tips) when a burning pain seared up through my heel and all of a sudden I could barely stand. I tried in vain to hobble back to my car but had to sit down on three different benches along the way. It took me over an hour to journey the quarter mile back. I'm generally slow on foot but not that slow!

There wasn't much I could do and I certainly wasn't going to put it on my medical records that I had a new condition 48 hours before my travel insurance kicked in, so I just had to grin and bear it over the next few days while my ankle and heel throbbed. I still packed all my running kit in my luggage – I was intending to run a 5k race whilst on holiday as well as take in some local run routes – and despite the searing pain I remained optimistic, like any good runner would.

Two days later, disembarking the plane after a nine-hour flight, I'm pretty sure the crew thought I was drunk as every time I tried to stand up my foot gave out beneath me and I'd yelp. At this point I didn't know it was Achilles tendinopathitisism and I probably should have visited the ER to rule out anything broken, but I wasn't going to risk slightly higher travel insurance premiums for my next holiday because of a tiny little issue like not being able to walk! I spent the entire two weeks hobbling around for a few minutes here and there before having to sit down again. My four-year-old niece Harley attempted to make my heel better with her Doc McStuffins medical playset and some wet paper towels – a well-known cure for most ailments. However, the damage was done.

Back home, I booked an appointment with Charlotte, my now long-suffering sports therapist for eight years, who promptly diagnosed what Doc McStuffins hadn't: Achilles tendonitis. It was four months before I was able to start running again.

I have wondered if it might have been one of the quickest onsets of an injury in a new runner, occurring just six weeks in. However, I recently watched a reality TV show where one of the cast signed up for a half marathon six weeks away and during her very first training run was determined to cover the full distance. As you might expect, she swiftly put an end to her training and left her forthcoming race hanging in the balance with all sorts of damage to her foot and limbs. No one told her about potential injuries as a new runner, not even the more accomplished runner who accompanied her on that first outrageous training run.

I suspect very few readers will be entirely injury free – so let's play a game of Injury Bingo! The rules are very simple. Just grab your dabber and dab off any injury you've sustained since you started running. There are no prizes. Just tears, probably.

INJURY BINGO			
Calf strain	Meniscal tear	Bursitis	Runner's knee
Morton's neuroma	Achilles tendonitis	Lost toenail(s)	Broken femur
IT band syndrome	Shin splints	Arse over Tit AKA 'The Jane'	Stress fracture
Anterior Compartment Syndrome	Grazed knee	Ran into a post AKA 'The Simon'	Stung by a wasp/bee mid-run
Plantar fasciitis	Faceplanted the pavement AKA 'The Joy'	Shredded nipples	Broken wrist
Torn hamstring	Broken ribs	Sprained ankle	Broken toe

<u>Injury bingo scoring</u>

No full line: Pah, you've barely scraped the surface of running injuries. Amateur!

A full line in any direction: Nice work! You're on a roll but there's plenty more to come.

Multiples lines in any direction: Impressive! You've spent more time on the bench than running.

Full house: Congratulations! You have achieved the highest status of injured runner and there is nothing left to achieve. Skill McGill!

When it comes to running injuries, it's one thing to be the cause of your own problems; for example, you ran too hard, for too long, too quickly and ended up with a near-ruptured Achilles tendon for four months. Who even does that?

However, it's another thing entirely when someone else causes you an injury that affects your running. I've seen numerous runners taken down by a dog that has found itself forced into running when all it wants to do is go and sniff a lamp post. Some dogs love running and some owners are skilled and experienced at taking those dogs for a run. Some dogs do not want to run and some owners are crap at controlling them on a lead.

Last week, at parkrun, I had to stop mid-run and grab a dog who had escaped his collar due to the owner savagely pulling the lead so hard while the dog resisted.

This week, I had to do the same thing with the same

dog and owner. One more time and I'm not giving the dog back!††

Another hazard I witnessed recently was a poor child on a scooter at parkrun. His dad had positioned him firmly in the centre of hundreds of runners, with the little one well below the eyeline of most people around him. The klaxon went and his dad sped off, and in his rush to keep up with his speedster dad, he found himself tangled in his scooter and taking down six or seven runners around him. When I reached the child, his dad was a hundred metres away, oblivious to the fact that his seven-year-old was on the floor crying and scared whilst shocked runners were picking gravel out of their knees. It was really upsetting for the child and at best frustrating for those who tripped over him; at worst it was dangerous for them – broken bones, head injuries and the like can happen in even the smallest of tumbles and this one involved metal and wheels.

The worst incident, at the hands of another, was Stuart's pre-race 'canning', which occurred the night

---

†† Oh my goodness, I had long finished this chapter, but I had to come back to tell you – it happened again! For the third time, I witnessed the same runner dragging the poor dog along. Once again it escaped its collar but this time it ran back towards the start line as the runner called after it but made little attempt to follow. Five or so minutes later the runner passed me, minus their dog. I can only hope they left him with a non-runner as it was far too hot for him to have been put back in the car – and surely they didn't just leave him loose and alone while they carried on running?

before one of his London Marathon attempts. The whole family were casually walking along a street in London, on our way to carb-load at our favourite pre-race Italian restaurant, when a lout in a loutish car with loutish mates threw a full, unopened can of beer out of the window directly towards us. It's a despicable person who aims to hurt another human being in such a way – but surely only a true moron would waste beer in the process.

Out of six of us, the beer can hit Stuart.

On his foot.

Fifteen hours before the London Marathon.

Talk about bad injury luck!

Thirty minutes later, we were sitting around our table at Jamie's Italian, eating rustic breads with oil and vinegar, while Stuart wrapped his foot in tea towels and ice kindly donated by Jamie's representatives in the kitchen!

The next day, despite having a foot the size of a balloon, Stuart did go on to complete the full marathon. The day after that, he went on to get a stern telling off from his sports therapist for running with such a bad injury.

While I was writing this chapter, I asked my running friends to share their running injuries with me. I expected to find myself with a list of the common injuries we've all heard of and probably already dabbed off in the game of Injury Bingo earlier: torn hamstring, Achilles tendonitis, sprained ankle, shin splints and so on.

Instead, what I got was a list of the most bizarre mishaps ever to happen to a runner – and it was more than I ever knew I needed to hear from them! What I had forgotten is that these are real runners and they don't just get the textbook injuries, they are out there finding the obscure and, if I'm honest, hilarious (although maybe not at the time) injuries.

Everyone had something truly brilliant to share, but once again my friend Daniel stole the show with numerous bizarre and baffling running injuries, many of which would bring tears to your eyes just hearing about. I know you're probably hoping I'll share the details, but I've decided not to as I think it's very possible he will write his autobiography one day soon and I don't want there to be any spoilers. It will be a fantastic read!

Instead, let's start with Jane. Jane tried to answer her phone mid-run and ploughed into a lamppost. I myself have walked into a lamppost (in full view of the always busy A45 highway) but I've never hit one at speed, which I imagine is equally as painful as it is embarrassing.

Simon and Dave both told me about running, crotch-first, into 'safety bollards'. The irony!

Kerrie seemed to win the people's vote during this discussion about bizarre running injuries when she told us about the time she tripped over a squirrel. Yes, a squirrel. On a picturesque route through St Albans, said squirrel came from nowhere, at speed, and he and

Kerrie collided. Kerrie squealed. The squirrel squealed. It sounds like the squirrel was actually more badly injured than Kerrie in this collision, based on the flailing around she says it did afterwards.

Marie explained about the time she was running on a treadmill and flew off at speed. Too embarrassed to do anything else, she hopped back onto the dreaded running machine and carried on to the end of the programme. It was only after Marie finished her workout that she noticed the bleeding and the dent in her shin – which is still present to this day. Also to this day, she now uses the safety clips religiously when on the treadmill.

Nicola, who kindly wrote the Polar Night Race Report for this book, was reminded of the time she tripped on a tree root mid-run and hurt her left shoulder. Like many of us, she wasn't going to let a little thing like that stop her from running and promptly went off for a run the following day. Unfortunately, she did the exact same thing (although I don't know if it was the same tree root) and, clearly displeased with the asymmetry of the previous day's injury, this time she hurt her right shoulder. I believe she rested on the third day!

Ian shared with me a gory photo of the time he didn't see the barbed wire that was obscured by some deep mud on his trail run. Not only does Ian have the photo as a reminder, he also has the scars.

A close contender to Kerrie for the most bizarre incident is Terry, although his was more of a near-miss than anything and luckily no injury was sustained, as I suspect it may have been a bad one had things gone the other way. Terry was running on a wintery day, dressed all in white as he thought it would aid visibility, and ended up coming very close to being run over by a snowplough.

Ok, let's have just one of Daniel's bizarre injury stories! Trying to escape a goring from a bull whilst running through its field, Daniel found himself heading towards a barbed wire fence. He had no choice but to jump it and, luckily, on this occasion he cleared it with space to spare (unlike the time he grabbed a barbed wire fence mid-run and the barbs went all the way through his hand). Unfortunately, there was a ditch on the other side of the fence, filled with stinging nettles that Daniel flew straight into upon clearing the barbed wire. He required a hefty dose of post-run anti-histamines to settle the head-to-toe swelling.

After lots of chit chat amongst our bizarrely injured runners, the tales eventually drew to a close – because there was simply nothing left that could conceivably happen to a runner. They had covered everything, from tripping over a squirrel to losing battles with barbed wire. The final offering came from Martyn, a clubmate who I have yet to meet properly but whose book *Accidental Ironman* I referred back to repeatedly whilst writing this book. Mostly to reassure myself that it was OK to use the occasional swear word! Martyn (or Shitclown, as he once refers to himself in his book whilst discussing what his *Gladiator* name might be) quietly and understatedly shared one single photograph to sum up his own ridiculous injury and provide a stark warning to other runners. The warning being:

"Wear sunscreen."

Now, I feel like that's been said by someone before, but Martyn clearly didn't heed the advice.

Looking at the photo, you could be forgiven for thinking he is wearing a sweater with a bold, geometric print in garish – but probably cool if you are young – colours. What you are actually looking at is a shirtless Martyn whose sunburn is so extreme and shining so brightly that I have to assume the photograph was taken by an A&E doctor. Martyn's wry smile in the photograph suggests he is actually quite proud of his extensive race-day toasting and, given what I've gleaned about his personality from *Accidental Ironman*, I think I've made a fair assessment that he suffered.

Although not an injury or niggle as such, there is one thing that affects most runners from time to time and that is the loss of mojo. Or, in some extreme cases, a serious loss of mojo. If you're lucky enough not to have experienced it, basically it's when you just can't be arsed to run. It's not when you're having one of those one-off, lazing-on-the-couch type evenings where it's just too cold outside to run. It's when you give up all desire for running and nothing can convince you to get out there. It's quite common in the come-down following a marathon. After mine, I felt I'd worked so hard for months and then, with nothing on the books to exert myself for, what began as a 'well-earned rest' somehow evolved into my love of running dying off entirely. I was still buzzing from having run the marathon but I had no interest in lacing up my shoes for the foreseeable future.

From speaking to running club mates I half knew to expect it, so I just rode out the time and ultimately it wore off when someone suggested the runners from our club all wear their London Marathon T-shirts to parkrun a few weeks later to celebrate our achievement. We were also to bring our medals along for a sort of impromptu community show-and-tell (even though, as usual, no asked to see or hear!). Of course, I wasn't going to miss the chance to show off my London Marathon medal and then once there, running a sunny 5k with my friends, I realised I still enjoyed running and instantly became eager to sign up for another race. Not another marathon, but a 10k or something.

If you are having an extreme flare-up of lost mojo there might not be much you can do. Just sit tight and the desire will come back. If you're almost there and just need that last push to rediscover yours, here are 20 of my favourites things you can do to pep yourself up.

1) Start easy and just go for a walk. Make sure you Strava it!

2) Buddy up and find someone else in your club or community who is feeling the same way and would be happy to join you on a comeback.

3) Start Couch to 5K. (I can recommend Sarah Millican as your coach – she always asks if you're doing OK pet!)

4) Sign up for a race. Even if you feel reluctant, get one on the books. If you have a favourite past race, sign up for it again and start a tradition.

5) Treat yourself to some new trainers or kit. You deserve it!

6) Create a running music playlist and then go test it out. At the top of mine right now is *Dancing in The Dark* by Bruce Springsteen AKA The Boss. It totally fires me up for running!

7) Sign up for parkrun, return to parkrun, choose a new parkrun to try, or sign up to volunteer. The community spirit was all I needed to get running again.

8) Change the time you run i.e. if you normally run at night, try the morning instead. Saying that, I myself can't run in the morning (except once when I did a sunrise 5k at 5am). The thought of getting out of bed to run is too horrific, even though I'm pretty much a morning person anyway.

9) Plan a new route and/or try a new distance. As above, a change is as good as a rest and some different scenery or a new challenge might inspire you.

10) Do some strength work. If you really aren't going to run right now, maybe see if you can get yourself run-fit for when you do return. You know you'll never do strength work again once you restart running, so get some in the bank now!

11) Get the family involved if they don't already run. They might really enjoy it and you can impart wisdom on those wet-behind-the-ears newbies, which is a runner's dream!

12) Adopt a new runner. Do you have a non-runner friend who'd like to get started and can benefit from your expertise?

13) PUB RUN! Get some mates together and run to and from the pub, stopping there of course for a few mid-run refreshments! (NB This will also work with cafes, chippies etc.)

14) Add in some drills (reps, hills, lampposts etc.) to an otherwise straight run. When I'm lacking mojo, I find it less daunting to do a short run with some drills thrown in than a long run, plodding away mile after mile.

15) Read a running book. I really like *Running Like a Girl* by Alexandra Heminsley and also this book you're reading right now!

16) Look back over your old race medals and photos for nostalgia. It's bound to remind you why you fell in love with running in the first place.

17) Change your focus. Running is generally good

for your overall health – so the end goal doesn't always need to include being fast, running far or racing. Sometimes just being fit, healthy and outdoors is enough of a goal.

18) Reward yourself! Maybe a little counter-productive and probably not what any of the legit running books would suggest but plan a reward (cake? wine? pizza?) and enjoy it after you tick off that first run back. NB It's totally OK if it's a small run and a big cake.

19) Watch the movie *Run Fatboy Run*. I decided I was going to run a marathon whilst watching this film, so who knows, it may inspire you to get back out running!

20) I don't have a 20th suggestion but a list of 19 felt a bit scrappy and unfinished.

I have spent most of my running life harbouring an injury (I mentioned my dodgy left side), probably all connected to that initial injury at the beginning of my journey. I have had just about every running-related condition or injury you can imagine, including three separate surgeries, all on that bloody left side. It's a wonder I don't run in circles! Aside from the injuries, though, I seem to be plagued by animal-related attacks in my sporting life. I'm not the only one; I recently spotted on Strava that my friend had titled her morning run 'Vicious Canadian goose on the loose. PB.'

This time last year I was running in the glorious

summer sunshine and a stripy, buzzing creature stung me on the face. I didn't even want to run that night; I forced myself to go out because the weather was lovely and we should all make the most of summer because we spend all winter moaning about the cold, blah blah blah. I still can't run down the road where it happened, Essex Close (or Sex Close, as someone changed it to when I was at primary school. It wasn't me, I should add; I just remember it being funny even though I wasn't 100% sure why).

I was running along, mentally writing my Instagram post about what a summery goddess of a runner I was, and how I was #blessed, when I was hit with an excruciating pain just below my eye. A wasp got me! It had me in tears – and I like to think I have a fairly strong pain threshold. Unfortunately, the sting wasn't the worst of it, and I had a very severe allergic reaction and swelling around my eyes. The entire left side of my face ballooned (again with the left side of my body!), so much so that I couldn't run parkrun the next day – I'm a path drifter as it is without loss of vision in one eye – so I volunteered instead. I will use this passage of the book to publicly offer my apologies to those runners who missed out on a PB that day because they either a) slowed down to get a morbidly curious look at my grotesque face or b) took a wide line to get as far away from me as possible. Either way, you all lost precious seconds.

It's quite unfortunate that at the same time my eye ballooned, I was also harbouring a foot injury that was causing me to limp (so I should never have been running parkrun that day anyway, but I had planned to, pre-sting) *and* I had an ear infection that left me struggling to hear. I think the name Quasimodo was shouted out by one or two runners (or fifty), but then again, I couldn't hear properly, so who knows?

On another occasion, I was stalked for potential attack by a large bird of prey during the Cotswold Hilly 100 race. Now, I'm not a bird expert but I think it was a bald eagle. Majestic but menacing. I know bald eagles are not native to this country but I think possibly this one was on vacation.

I was a few miles into my 10-mile leg of the race and I had already slogged up (but somehow not down) about 15 hills. Yes, the sweat was mixing with my sunscreen and burning my eyes but I still had clear enough vision to realise there was a ferocious-looking bird circling above me. Over the next few miles, it would hover over me then fly on ahead to sit in a tree and glare down at me. As I passed each time, it would circle overhead (no doubt mocking my slow place) and then re-perch in the next tree, staring. Waiting.

To my horror, it would occasionally take a small dip down towards me before retreating when a car or another runner came along. I recall there being an area called Slaughter on my leg of the race and imagined the newspaper headline the following day would read something like 'Slaughtered in Slaughter. Eagle decapitates runner' and they'd probably use the worst running photo of me ever. I don't know what his

227

agenda was that day, be it casual thuggery or something more sinister, but I did survive unscathed. Luckily, it hadn't made its move by mile 10, where I handed over the baton to the next runner and jumped into the safety of my car. The bird became her problem at that point. I haven't seen her since actually but I'm sure she's fine. Probably.

My lovely friend Sam provides the race report to end this chapter on running injuries. To my knowledge, Sam has never been attacked mid-run by a bald eagle, but at the end of the Edinburgh Marathon she did find out that she'd fallen foul of the sun, which is something that happens to most of us in the summer running months. I'm usually so red in the face through exertion that it takes me a good few hours to notice that I forgot to apply sunblock before the run. Generally, Sam had an injury-free race in Edinburgh, so this is one of those race reports where there's very little connection to the chapter content. Interestingly, when I asked my running friends for race reports that involved injuries, no one offered anything. Like me, they probably don't want to be reminded of their injury-plagued races when they have so many other good ones to share.

Race Report
Sam's Edinburgh Marathon

We travelled to Edinburgh by car, a 7-hour journey and the equivalent distance of almost 13 marathons – 338 miles, I think. It was my second marathon, just over four and a half years since my first and the only one since I had been diagnosed with and treated for the big C.

We stayed in Crammond, a picturesque place with water and boats. It's also excellent if you want a parkrun the day before the marathon as there is one just a few minutes away from the accommodation in which we stayed, by the water's edge.

The lead up to the marathon by the organisers was incredibly informative and it really prepared you for the race, allowing you to book buses from the park and rides on the outskirts of the city and back from the finish (you cannot park at the finish). It gave detail about the course and what to expect on the day. The race number arrived in good time and I felt ready to go.

The day of the marathon arrived. The weather forecast said it was going to be cool and cloudy; perfect conditions, but it couldn't have been more wrong. While the wait to start was almost cold, within minutes of crossing the start line at 10.21am the sun appeared and it warmed up very quickly, reaching temperatures in the mid-20s. I had prepared for almost everything except the heat.

The start area was overlooked by the hills and it was a beautiful backdrop to await the beginning of the race. Plenty of portaloos were provided and lorries to put your bags into, which were then driven to the finish.

The course took you through the city, past many of the famous sites and out towards the coast. The start was downhill but once out of the city you began to climb. After about 6 miles the course took you along the seafront and past families enjoying the by now very warm weather. One kind little girl offered me an ice lolly at 7 miles but I politely refused. By 16 miles, I would have snapped her hand off!

I was running for Breast Cancer Now and had my charity vest on. The race numbers had been printed with the runner's name on. I lost count of the number of people who called my name and congratulated me on running for my chosen charity. The support along the course until about 16 miles was amazing. The course continued uphill, partly following the coast and partly inland.

The race organisers had made sure there were plenty of toilets as well as water and gel stations. It was so hot that I took on almost an entire bottle of water at every station after the 7-mile mark, even crossing over to the other side of the road to grab water at one point.

One very kind gardener had directed their sprinkler onto the pavement so we could run through the cooling spray, which made us all very happy.

Just after 16 miles, the road was divided into two with the finishers on the right-hand side and the slower runners (me; I wasn't alone though) on the left. I expected to find this demoralising but it was far from it. In both the marathons that I have competed in I have experienced a real dip at 16 miles and I found it so encouraging to be able to observe how much the faster runners were also struggling; I could fully appreciate that a marathon really is an incredibly tough challenge. I think when you have been running a while you can say, "Oh, it's only a marathon," but we'd do well to never forget how far that is and a number of the spectators recognised this by saying if it were easy we'd all be doing it. Once the course split into two I also recognised the three runners who I'd had a really good chat to before the race and they smiled at me, which really spurred me on.

I found the 16-19 mile stretch really hard. At 19 miles you go into an off-road section around some fields and remote houses and then you turn back towards the finish in Musselburgh. Unfortunately, this is an area where the spectators do not venture and there are few people nearby – but the view looking out to sea is fantastic. The course continues back down through the same two villages you run through on your way out to the 19-mile point. By now the weather was, thankfully, a bit cooler.

At 22 miles my watch died, helpfully, so after that I did not know how much further I had to run or what the time was. I called out to someone who was going into a local shop to ask them.

Then before too long the glorious finish was within sight and almost within reach. The finish funnel/area itself is quite long and lined with iron barriers with banners with the EMF logo on them. There is a sharp bend to the left until you run through the finish. All along this area spectators were banging their hands on the barriers, which was so uplifting and just what you needed after a 26.1-mile run in the heat!

My daughter was an especially welcome sight in the finish village. I mounted the podium for a finish photo and we headed off to find a taxi, both too exhausted to walk to the bus. My finish time was texted to me shortly after I left the race village and I was extremely pleased to learn that I had achieved a PB.

After my bath that evening I discovered I was really sunburnt, but I was so pleased that I'd completed my challenge of running the Edinburgh Marathon and in the process raised £1,000 for Breast Cancer Now. I would thoroughly recommend it to anyone wanting a city marathon; however, don't believe them when they say it is a flat course as it's simply not true.

Chapter Ten
The Joy of parkrun

My very first goal in this chapter is to reassure everyone that I understand that:

1) parkrun is written as a single word
2) parkrun is spelled with a lower-case p

I just wanted to get that out of the way, right off the bat.

Misspelling the word 'parkrun' can be a contentious issue and I've seen Facebook threads descend into chaos following someone writing 'Park Run' and someone else insulting them over it. If you feel strongly enough to explain the situation to someone, that's totally fine – as long as you're not a jerk about it! Imagine joining one of the friendliest and most inclusive communities around the world and then belittling a stranger on the internet who may have just been a victim of an overly-enthusiastic autocorrect!

My own fear that I would make a grammatical error in this chapter is the reason it is only a few pages long. Minimise the risk! At least 10 times my spell checker has automatically changed parkrun to park run and I'm terrified that the proof reader is going to change parkrun at the beginning of a sentence to a P and I'll hear about it in the online book reviews!

parkrun themselves explain the reason behind

their lowercase branding as 'the little p mentality' – a representation of the simplicity and inclusion of parkrun events and the ethos of the organisation. It is a symbol of how parkrun is meant to be fun, friendly and inclusive.

I saw a post on social media recently where someone asked, "What is parkrun all about?" and one helpful responder simply wrote "Running."

Well, they're not wrong really and for some runners it's really that basic. They run. They run at parkrun on a Saturday. That is all.

For many though, there is much more depth to parkrun and it touches on the social, emotional and spiritual aspects of human wellbeing.

So, there are really two descriptions of parkrun, the one you get if you Google it:

Q: What is parkrun?

A: parkrun is a weekly 5-kilometre timed event for runners, walkers and volunteers that takes place on a Saturday.

And the one you get if you ask a passionate parkrunner:

Q: What is parkrun?

A: Oh it's fantastic! You get to catch up with friends, meet new people, clear your head, release any anxieties, forget about the real world and get some time away from the kids… You can have a coffee and some cake afterwards, there's usually a selfie frame, which is fun, we give everyone a big cheer when they reach milestones or are celebrating an occasion, you can bring your dog or your pushchair, there's lots of cheering and the volunteers are so supportive. You can do it at your own pace, there's no pressure, it's all very inclusive. You can even walk it. You'll meet like-minded people and travel to interesting destinations. Oh yeah, so it's a weekly 5-kilometre timed event for runners, walkers and volunteers that takes place on a Saturday.

I like that in the people's definition, the actual matter of running comes last after all the social interactions and fun stuff!

For me, I think the joy of parkrun comes from the fact that it is so diverse, in all aspects. Lined up at the front are the fastest runners – there's usually some jostling and stiff competition between them. They get a bit competitive. Then, if you travel all the way down the line to where you'll usually find me, you've got walkers, injured runners, pushchair runners and plenty of dogs. A few dogs and pushchairs in the hands of some very fast runners do make it further up the field but largely they stay at the back. There are runners who are super-svelte and gazelle-like and the rest of us meagre mortals who might be a little less toned in places. There are runners of all ethnicities, cultures and backgrounds. I'm always very impressed by one older lady from the local Indian community who runs in very heavy clothing appropriate to her culture. I was particularly pleased to see my GP running a few weeks ago as the practice now prescribes parkrun in some cases of anxiety, stress and depression. The idea behind this is that taking part in an event like parkrun gives patients the opportunity to socialise, make friends and be part of a community, all of which is great for general health and mental wellbeing, not to mention the physical benefits that taking part can have on the body and patient health.

If you visit your local parkrun frequently, you tend to see the same faces at the same point in the start funnel and that's why it's a great place to meet friends. I know that most weeks I can start at one end of the funnel and pinpoint the exact position of most of my running friends for a quick hello as I make my way ever further towards the back! This is true except in the case of those of my running friends who are eternal parkrun tourists – that is, they enjoy the experience of visiting a different parkrun around the country, and the world, each week. My friend Ian and his children Iona and Ewan take on a different parkrun most Saturdays, exploring new areas to run in and, perhaps most importantly, rating the post-parkrun breakfasts on their YouTube channel *A Little Adventure with Ian & Family*. Iona recently ran her 80th parkrun at her 80th different venue, which is quite an achievement for someone so young.

One of my friends ran in his 250th different parkrun location recently, which is also incredibly impressive – but he's a grown-up, so Iona wins!

I'm sure there are people out there who don't know parkrun exists, never mind that 250 exist. In fact, in the 20 countries that parkrun operates, there are almost

1,700 different events. I have taken part in 14 different parkruns, so I have a way to go if I want to do them all (I don't!) but I have, however, just completed my 100th parkrun, which is a recognised milestone rewarded with a very nice black running top to mark the occasion. Well, I say rewarded; you have to pay for it but it's worth the few pounds to let people know you've joined the respected 100 Club! The best bit about this particular milestone is that the next one isn't until 250, so when I am out running, wearing my 100 T-shirt, no one knows if I've done 101 parkruns or 249! (Full disclosure, at the time of writing it's 101.)

Most of my parkruns have been at my 'home' parkrun, which is Coventry. Coventry parkrun was started by my clubmate and friend Jason back in 2010 and has since held over 550 events. I think it's fair to say that Jason and his family have been there for almost all of them, either directing, volunteering, or running. Jason's mum, Phyll, has just recently completed her 500th parkrun. That's over 10 years of Saturday mornings spent careering around a local park. I use the word 'careering' here with great joy since the dictionary definition is *moving swiftly and in an uncontrolled way* and that's very 'Phyll'. It's not a style most runners aspire to, and indeed no running manual will guide you towards this, but Phyll is one of us – she's a real runner who makes her own rules about what running and parkrun should be like. Just this past Saturday, she came 'careering' past me, ringing a bell – it was Christmas, but still, the woman ran an entire parkrun with a bell! If you are feeling inspired by Phyll's 500 parkruns, I think it's even more incredible to note that she also has over 180 volunteer credits to her name. What a parkrun legend you are, Phyll! (And that's the nicest I will ever be to you, so you might want to frame this page!)

I did ask Phyll the other day if she has nothing better to do on a Saturday morning. She replied that the only reason she actually comes at all is to heckle me whilst I run…

Very occasionally will you find Jason heckling you at the finish line, as he is very much his mother's son, but mostly the *unofficial* volunteer role of 'heckler' is saved for the brilliant Mark – I have yet to cross the Coventry parkrun finish line when Mark is on duty and not be told to do another lap because "That last one was crap!" All in good humour, I must stress – we all know he only says it to people he really likes. And if he gets too out of line, Carol, his wife, is never far away to take a swipe at his head!

At the last count before the pandemic, Coventry parkrun was attracting circa 900 participants each week and even now, with numbers a little lower following the pandemic, plus the opening of numerous nearby parkruns, it is still an impressive sight watching 400-500 runners file around the War Memorial Park just after 9am every Saturday. Keeping them safe, we are quite lucky to have great regulars who volunteer each week. One corner along the route is fondly known as 'Bryan's Corner' on account of the lovely gentleman who stands there each week high-fiving and cheering on runners. Bryan has been one of Coventry parkrun's most regular volunteers, having racked up nearly 300 volunteer credits, and we all look forward to his welcome cheers at the end of the long, uphill slog to his corner.

Another great feature at Coventry is that the race briefing is regularly interpreted into British Sign Language – parkrun is so inclusive and this is a great example of how we embrace that.

When it comes to parkrun, I am quite a simple girl. I rarely travel to other events, usually only ticking off different parkruns if I'm going to be nearby on a Saturday for some other reason. Many of my tourist parkruns have been in Wales while I was on holiday, a few have been in London on marathon weekend and all the rest have been in Coventry or very local to Coventry. I have visited one overseas parkrun, in Iowa, USA. After travelling 4,500 miles, I arrived to find the run director was from Nottingham, 50 miles from my hometown, and the first runner I spoke to turned out to be from London. It was the smallest parkrun I've ever visited, with about 20 runners and volunteers in total, but it had the same vibe as any of the bigger ones I've been to. Every runner got their well-deserved cheers and we visitors were made to feel like we'd been going for years!

One thing I hear about but never partake in are the parkrun 'quests' some runners go on – at the time of writing, I don't even know if 'quest' is the correct word but I hear runners talking about going to get their 'Alphabet' or their 'NENDY' and that sounds to me like they're on a quest. I think I know enough from talking to people that the Alphabet Challenge involves completing parkruns that begin with all the letters of the alphabet from A to Z. Except X, as there isn't a parkrun beginning with X (although I suppose you could apply some liberal interpretation and maybe run Exmouth?). However, I genuinely don't know what NENDY means, despite hearing it almost weekly.

Excuse me while I go and find out…

…OK, that clears it up. I have discovered that going to do your NENDY parkrun is going to do your Nearest Event Not Done Yet. Plus I just read on the parkrun blog (https://blog.parkrun.com/) that they do use the word 'quest' when talking about such activities!

So, for me, my current NENDY is Warwick Racecourse. Once I've ticked that off, it will be Babbs Mill, then Rugby. I can see how this can become addictive. You'll always be chasing your NENDY in this game!

While Googling NENDY, I also found out about:

- The Compass Club, where participants seek to do parkruns beginning with North, South, East and West. For example, Northampton parkrun, Eastbourne parkrun and so on.
- The 'The' tour, where participants aim to visit all 12 parkruns that currently begin with the

word 'The'. They'll have to head to the likes of Australia, South Africa and beyond to complete this challenge, so it's definitely one for the most dedicated!

- A particularly whimsical quest named The Pirate Club – you'll need to complete seven parkruns beginning with the letter C and one starting with the letter R (as in seven 'seas' and an arrrrggghhh…)

If you are keen on parkrun tourism or quests, you can find details of many more of them here: blog.parkrun.com/uk/tag/parkrun-tourism-series.

While some people are out there ticking off hundreds of parkruns, it's clearly not for everyone. My brother-in-law Simon has done one parkrun, and one parkrun only. He didn't hate it; he just felt no real desire to do another one and the longer time goes on, the more he revels in telling people how he has only ever done it once and intends to keep the not-running-parkrun streak going. It's a slightly easier streak to sustain than that of my friends who are aiming not to miss a parkrun all year (and longer in some cases!).

While I'm here, talking about Simon and his one run, I have to quickly mention my friend Lindsay (because I told her I would!). She just reminded me that she came for a run with me once. And only once. She has never laced up and run again since… I'm trying not to take it personally.

I'm interested to see if either Simon or Lindsay can indeed keep their never-running-again streak going!

One of my fellow parkrunners is the wonderful Brenda, who organised our Virtual London Marathon event. Brenda is married to one of the Daves in the club. Or she's married to someone called Dave who's not in the club but just shares his name with a club member. We're never quite sure who the real Dave is and actually, we've never seen either Brenda's Dave or the other Dave who shares his name in the same room. Brenda kindly shared the following race report with me. It's an interesting one as the race takes place, in part, in a tunnel! It's not parkrun related – again, I didn't get any race reports that I could link to this chapter – but it does mention 'parkrun', so this is one of my tenuously linked race reports!

Race Report
Brenda's Mersey Tunnel 10k

My daughter Hannah had booked to do the Mersey Tunnel 10k, so I decided to take the opportunity to visit her and also do the race myself.

The race morning started off chilly and we were happy to finally see the sun breaking through as we stood waiting at the start line. It had been very straightforward getting to the start, two double decker buses were waiting to take our luggage to the finish line in the Wirral and there was an adequate number of portaloos!

The race began on time and I was literally in the Kingsway Tunnel before I knew it. The tunnel started with a decline and it was easy to get carried away. It then levelled out the deeper we got. I passed the 1 kilometre and 2-kilometre markers before finding the route became much steeper. All through the tunnel, there were shouts of "Oggy! Oggy! Oggy!" and the sound of trainers hitting the road – all of this brought back brilliant memories of the Great North Run, which I have previously taken part in.

The 3-kilometre marker came into view right as I exited the tunnel before a swift turn to the left took me up the steepest part of the route. This was also where I found the first water station.

I reached the Wirral and turned into an industrial estate, from which point the route was flat. I was soon running along the River Mersey, with the long promenade laid out in front of me. I took the time to look over my shoulder and caught sight of the Liver Building. By now, the kilometre markers were passing swiftly, and I settled into a comfortable, steady pace, taking the time to enjoy the views of both the Wirral and the Liverpool waterfront.

The support on route was quite lean, but the pockets of supporters that were there as well as the marshals were all very good.

I reached 9 kilometres and I could see a fort-type building, which I later found out was Fort Perch Rock. It was an impressive-looking building that I also thought was the finish line, but no, there was still a left turn to do!

After the turn, the finish line came into view and although my number one fan, The Other Dave Lee, was for once not able to be there, I knew my daughter Hannah would be. Despite her saying, "I will stay with you, Mum," and "I think I am going to have to walk most of it," I knew her young legs and netball fitness would carry her through the race – and after the first 100 metres she had long gone from my view.

It was a lovely supportive finish and I was so pleased that I felt strong and in control of my race. There was no PB but how I had run the race mattered so much more to me and when I discovered that my last mile was my fastest, I was overjoyed. This had never happened before and I was hoping that when I told my running friend, Lesley Keighley, she would be proud of me. She has always told me to keep something in the bag for the finish!

My medal was put around my neck by a lovely lady. I always think this is such a nice touch, rather than just being handed your medal. I then received what seemed like an endless amount of post-race goodies and, finally, a winter training race T-shirt.

I soon found Hannah. She had finished in under an hour, so was delighted – I am very proud of her! She was, however, feeling discomfort in her hip, so she decided to go for a massage. By now the sun had gone and it was cold again, so I went off to get us each a much-needed hot drink and a cheese toastie. I would imagine on a warm day people would hang around and celebrate their success but people were soon making their way home because of the cold.

In order to get back to Liverpool, we had to catch the train. It was a short walk to the station and there were lots of runners on the train. This brought back memories of my train journey home last year after the London Marathon. It is always really lovely just seeing everyone with their medals and talking about their race. We were soon back in Liverpool and home to see how DIY Dave was getting on boarding the loft! Our daughter's house needs had been priority over being my number one fan, LOL!

There were two lovely moments during the race that stand out, one right at the start when someone shouted, "Hi Massey, I always see one of you!" and then later in the race when someone shouted, "Hi Coventry, welcome to Merseyside."

So, to sum up, this was a really nice race, it has the potential to be very fast, and there was a good medal and T-shirt, and plenty of goodies too. I am lucky that I have free accommodation in Liverpool but is it worth a night's hotel stay just for a 10K? Well, if you combine it with a bit of parkrun tourism at one of the Liverpool parkruns or a trip around Liverpool enjoying the many tours, museums, shops, bars and restaurants, then yes, it could be part of a really enjoyable running weekend. For me, two things made it very special: getting to do a race with my daughter, and being the first Massey runner over the finish line!

Chapter Eleven
Don't Believe
Every Motivational Quote
You Read on the Internet

In case you hadn't realised it, there's a lot of stuff on the internet. I think at this point in the history of the world wide web, you could Google 'running memes' today and still be scrolling through what's on offer this time next year. The trouble is that many, dare I say most of them, are empty, meaningless click-bait.

There are some comedy memes and quotes that I do like; for example, there's that one with a bear chasing a runner down a mountain accompanied by the tagline "Some days you can't find any motivation... Some days motivation finds you."

That one, I like. Who here wouldn't go for a quick run if a bear came up behind them?

Oh, and the one with four images of Shia LaBeouf crying, accompanied by the words "When all your friends are out running and you're just an injured piece of shit."

That one really speaks to me, as I go into my fourth year harbouring some sort of running injury!

I'm also a regular sharer of the Jason Bateman "The fuck you are" meme (from the movie *Identity Thief*) to acknowledge that whatever I say pre-race is unlikely to actually be the case once the klaxon goes. For example:

Me: "I'm recovering from an injury so I'm going to take this race sensibly."

My brain: "The fuck you are."

There are a few nuggets of genuinely motivational content out there on the internet if you look really carefully. For example:

"Everyone who runs is a runner."

YES! I like this one. No one should feel like they are not a runner because they don't cover as much distance as someone else, or because they don't enter races, or they aren't as fast as those who pass them. Everyone who runs is a runner. Preach!

"Running should never be a chore."

I also really like this one, not that I take it on board myself. I'm totally guilty of taking running so seriously that I forget why I'm doing it (which, by the way, is so I can eat all the French Fancies I like). I stop enjoying the social and fun runs and end up burning out and getting fed up with running. Then it takes me months to get my mojo back. It starts to become a vicious cycle. For the first few weeks after I get back into running, you'll hear me banging on about "I'm just enjoying running again" and "I'm so pleased to be back out running, no pressure" but before long, after another failed PB attempt, you'll be hearing how I "need a break from running" all over again. I'm stuck in an infinite loop.

I know most everyday runners share memes and motivational quotes with good intentions. Most of us just enjoy the sentiment; it speaks to us in some way and we want to share it with our running friends in case it encourages them or helps them overcome a running hurdle. That's nice. It's the pseudo-motivational nonsense shared by influencers who are just trying to get their likes up that I have less time for. The ones who don't actually have any real message to share or, worse, have a message that is potentially quite damaging to runners. They have nothing valuable to offer other than to remind us of the overuse of Comic Sans in bad internet memes. I've picked some and shared them below.

Of course, I'm not trying to make anyone feel bad for sharing or believing in any of these, so if you get some value from them, who am I to judge? If these get you through a tough time or give you the will you need to complete a difficult race, that's great. You do you! But for anyone who feels they can be damaging or make you feel inadequate when you don't achieve the headiest heights of running, be sure to scroll past any memes or motivational quotes that suggest any of the following.

"Running... you may not always want to but if you make yourself do it, you'll always be glad you did."

The word 'make' gives me the jitters every time I see it in relation to running. Something like this is not motivational; it just accelerates disengagement. I suppose if you happen to be looking for the quickest way to make running a chore, this might be the motivational quote for you. It's probably not for you though if you're like me and have days when you don't feel like running because:

a) you're feeling lazy

b) the weather looks rubbish

c) you just want to sit on the sofa and eat six French Fancies in a row (even the gross chocolate ones)

d) all of the above

On these days, I **remind** myself of the benefits of running, i.e. physical, mental, emotional and social, plus all the bragging rights I will have on social media once I get back, but I never **force** myself to run, which is what this meme suggests is a helpful approach. The reminder of the benefits is usually enough to get me out the door but there are occasions when I still don't feel like running and on those days, I definitely shouldn't. I personally think it's far healthier to opt out of your run if you have genuine reasons for needing to stay in that day. As much as we often feel better after a run, it is not a cure-all for everything and everyone, all the time. If there's any chance your run is going to turn you into a monster, it's best to follow that classic mantra made famous during the COVID-19 pandemic: stay home, save lives!

"Your legs are not quitting, your heart is. Keep going."

This is a very sweet sentiment figuratively but it's literally not true. There have been times when I've desperately wanted to run on but my legs have been on fire and I've had to stop. It was nothing to do with my heart quitting – I'm fairly certain if my heart had been quitting, I probably wouldn't be writing this book right now! As runners, we are often conditioned to believe that stopping is not an option – that stopping is quitting and quitting is wrong.

Public Service Announcement (that I will in no way adhere to myself): If you really need to stop on a run, you can stop. It's not 'quitting'; it doesn't make you weak. It means you are sensible and are listening to your body.

"No matter how slow you go, you are still lapping everyone on the couch."

For me personally, this means nothing. I'm pretty confident that most of the people at home on their couch right now could get up and spank me around any run they like!

"If it's not hard, it's not worth it."

This one makes me mad! Why is it not worth it to go out for an easy, simple run that I enjoy, that gives me some energy and endorphins, which lets my body heal from the heavy training I've been doing, or gives me some quiet headspace and alone time? Why is it not worth it to go out and run with my friend who is a bit slower than I am, or my friend who doesn't go as far as I do? It might not be a hard run for me, but I certainly feel it's worth it to spend time with my friend, supporting their running. Do all the easy runs you like if that's what you enjoy or what works for you!

"The reason we race is not so much to beat each other, but to be with each other."

I love running with my friends – chatting, gossiping, moaning, putting the world to rights and so on – but I promise you, if a finish line comes into sight I am dropping them like a stone and they would do exactly the same to me. A few years ago, Jo and I ran Massey's flagship race together, The Tractor 10k, chatting and encouraging each other during the tough parts and repeatedly mugging to the race photographer over the three-lap course. I think he was just pretending to press the shutter button by the last lap!

Towards the end, I'd actually forgotten it was a race and as we turned the corner to the finish line, I was mid-sentence – something about baked potatoes, I think – when Jo kicked up a gear and made a break for the finish, leaving me for dust. You can actually see the whole process unfold in one of the official race photos – my head is turned towards Jo, my mouth is wide open, mid-sentence, and Jo is just drifting out of shot, out of focus, a red and white blur. You can see in the next photo that I put in a sprint myself but I didn't catch her. She'd had the element of surprise and given herself a two second head start, which was all she needed to drop me. In the finish line photo, she is doubled over with laughter!

There are two things that annoy me about that race:

1) That she beat me.

2) That I didn't think of going first.

No, make that three things…

3) That it resulted in a really ugly finish line photo of me.

Actually, it's four things…

4) That I am a total running hypocrite who, on any other day, will tell you it doesn't matter if someone beats you!

"If you can dream it, you can do it."

I can daydream right now about crossing the finish line of my next 10k in 32 minutes. I will never be able to do this. No amount of training and/or dreaming will ever enable me to do this.

"A short run is better than no run."

I don't believe in this at all. There are lots of occasions when no run is the best thing for you.

"I broke four toes this morning but I'll get a short run in. Better than nothing."

I think not!

I've been out on many runs that were just a mile here or a mile there, so I'm not saying short runs aren't important. They absolutely are if they are part of your training plan or if it's just what you feel you need to do that day. But if you are forcibly trying to squeeze in a run where you simply can't or forcing yourself to run when your body physically won't allow it, running will become an unpleasant chore that causes you more stress than it's worth. I reckon if you miss a run, you miss a run. Give yourself a break!

"If it doesn't challenge you, it doesn't change

you."

Oh please! Why can't we just enjoy running without it needing to be a constant challenge?

Also, I don't want to change, thanks very much! I'm willing to bet that the same influencer who shared this has also shared "Never change, you're amazing as you are."

"Learn to run when feeling the pain, then push harder."

I can't believe there's someone out there who thinks this is a healthy, motivational quote to share with other runners. Unlearn this! Pain is not something to ignore or believe you have to run through just to be a 'good' runner. As we discussed earlier, pain is not always a sign of chronic or serious damage – it manifests in various ways, to various degrees, some of which may not be a major cause for concern – but still, it shouldn't ever be ignored in the pursuit of pushing harder. Most of us will feel pain during a race and still press on to finish, that's just the runner's way, but we don't have to push harder; instead, we can slow down, take a walking break, visit the aid station etc. The above should not become a mantra that spurs us on and tells us to ignore pain; it's dangerous.

"Just run – pain is nothing compared to what it feels like to quit."

Again with the quitting. It's OK to 'quit', although I don't really think we need to assign that particular word to every occasion when we don't finish a run.

There are lots of reasons you might stop a run or renege on a training plan. If you've made a healthy, positive decision to pull out of a race, or maybe not even start the race at all, it's not quitting. And you would definitely not enjoy forcing yourself through it, only to be in pain later.

I've made this mistake many times, so I'm not virtue signalling here. I will probably make the same mistake again many times in the future. I've run and finished races knowing something wasn't right in my body but I've forced myself along, saying, "I'll just get through the last mile and then whatever it is, I'll deal with it later." I've gotten home, shared my 'success' on social media and Strava, proclaimed how amazing my run was, that it was tough but I kept going and finished it strong. Hurrah! What a running hero I am!

Then, when the little red notifications have stopped pinging through, all I'm left with is panic and fear about what damage I might have done. Why didn't I follow my own advice and stop? Why couldn't I be proud of myself for what I'd done up to the point I stopped and, what's more, be proud of myself for taking care of my body when it needed taking care of?

You know the answer: because I'm a runner and we don't practise what we preach!

"Pain is weakness leaving the body."

The most scientifically inaccurate thing I've ever read on the internet, ever. Which is saying something, because there is a lot of fake news out there.

Please note, the race reports ended in Chapter Ten as it was a nice round number that pleased me and the remaining chapters take a different format and are shorter. Just in case you still think I'm an amateur writer and just forgot to add one here… Oh, and I've reached my word count now, so I don't feel I need to try anymore!

Chapter Twelve
I Was Overtaken By...

There is a great moment in every race when you get a surge of confidence in your running ability. Despite your lack of training and a poorly chosen race-day breakfast, things seem to be going surprisingly well. You have life in your legs and air in your lungs and you feel capable of finishing the race strong and actually getting a decent finish line photo for once.

And then you are overtaken by a snail!

Not an actual snail, of course, but a runner wearing an oversized, elaborate snail costume who beats you over the line.

Or maybe you were passed by an actual snail?

For all but one person at any given time, there is always a better runner in the race. For me, there are lots of better runners and they often pass me dressed in costumes that would suffocate and consume me within minutes of the starting klaxon. With that in mind, I challenged my Instagram followers to finish the sentence "I was overtaken by…" and it turned out better than I ever imagined.

I've compiled a list of the best/weirdest responses.

I was overtaken by…

- A giant banana
- A runner wearing skinny jeans
- A man dressed as a condom

- Gritty – the extremely large fluffy mascot of National Hockey League team the Philadelphia Flyers
- The entire cast of the 70s children's puppet show Rainbow – that's Zippy, Bungle and George!
- A drag queen wearing one stiletto

I long to know what happened to the other stiletto!

- A parent with a double stroller, going uphill – a very steep hill
- A kayak… the route was incredibly flooded!
- A runner carrying a fridge on his back
- A caterpillar; that is, seven runners dressed in green fur and attached to one another

I myself was once passed in the London Marathon by a group of butterflies. Could it have been the same runners and they'd since metamorphosed?

- A couple dressed in life-sized matching giraffe costumes
- A heavily pregnant parent pushing another child in a stroller
- A giraffe aiming for the world record attempt at the tallest London Marathon costume

Giraffes seem to be a popular, and speedy, choice.

- The Jamaican bobsleigh team
- The Badger from Badgers 10k
- A 9-year-old at parkrun
- An inflatable dinosaur, a rhino, a gorilla, a bobsleigh team (they get around!), a Roman soldier, Superman, Superwoman, and a man

carrying a karaoke machine (many of us will know Karaoke Man!). By the way, this was all at the same race!

- A rhino

Another popular costume choice.

- Noddy, complete with his Noddy car
- The Honey Monster
- A person on a mobility scooter
- A bumble bee

At first, I thought this person was telling me that an actual flying insect beat them across the finish line but it turns out it was a runner dressed as a bumble bee "with a pathetic, lame buzz that sounded more like the noise a 99p handheld fan makes when the motor is burning out."

- Chewbacca
- A race walker

My friend Ian, who shared this one, also mentioned that he was once almost overtaken by "a turd" but he managed to take him at the finish! Glad to hear your race didn't go down the pan, Ian! Yes, I did just make that terrible toilet pun intentionally.

- Another rhino

Is this the same person going around beating everyone or is it lots of different rhinos?

- A man pushing two toddlers uphill in a double stroller… carrying a rucksack… wearing sandals
- A rhino named Julian

Finally, someone got the rhino's name!

- Two jacket potatoes

This is my favourite response because I can't understand a scenario where a jacket potato is a valid couples' running costume. I have to assume they had their reasons.

- A giant boob
- Dave Adams… just a guy I know called Dave Adams

I also know a Dave Adams! Could it be the same Dave Adams?

- A man wearing a thong
- Just lots and lots of other people
- Dogs, plural
- A runner in short shorts with a back pocket completely overloaded with gels, the weight of which kept pulling the shorts down to reveal his bottom. Right in my eyeline!
- A panto horse… not once, not twice but three times in the same race

Oh no you didn't! (I'm sorry, I had to. I kept trying not to type it, but the urge was too strong!)

- A very elderly runner telling me to "Keep going, you'll get there!"
- A spectator in very high heels who jumped onto the course to run with a friend through the finish
- A man smoking a cigarette
- Mr Blobby

Now, I know I've already said somewhere in this book (there are 70,000+ words, so forgive me for forgetting exactly where!) that it's OK to beat others in a race and it's OK to have others beat you because it's not a race against them, it's just a race against yourself and blah blah blah blah blah. Yes, I stand by that and yes, it's true, but it's not always true. It's only sometimes true. Do you know what I mean?

I mean that in real life, we runners seem to have 'fluctuating' or 'occasional' truths. In other words, there are things we repeatedly tell ourselves and other runners about running that we really believe at that particular point in time. Then the next week, day, or even the next hour – because we are quite fickle as a group – we will be unwavering in our belief that the opposite is true.

Case in point:

Me, recently preaching evangelically to my nervous friend on race day: "Just remember, someone has to come last and it's the taking part that counts. All that matters is you enjoy the race. It's not important whether you win or lose; just have a good time."

Also me, on the same race day, to my running bestie: "As long as I don't come last, I don't care. Oh my God, if I come last, I'll die. That would be the most embarrassing thing ever. Ever! If I come last, I'm never running again!"

Fickle.

And as you know, I have come dead last in a race

and it wasn't that bad. Everyone clapped a lot, which was nice.

Still, as much as we protest to others that it's totally OK, we often do feel embarrassed at the thought of being overtaken or coming last in a race. Recently, I was on holiday in South Wales and went out for a run along the Llanelli coast path. This was not a race, not even a parkrun. It was just a casual 5k run to enjoy the beautiful scenery and surroundings.

I was running along, happy and feeling at one with nature, when a younger runner came from behind and passed me on the narrow path. The second I saw her weave back in front of me, totally oblivious, unrelated, and uninterested in me or my running in any way whatsoever, it naturally became a race.

"Err who does she think she is, just passing me like that?"

I was only out for a slow, steady run to keep my injury recovery on plan but that went out of the window instantly. Quick as a flash, I picked up the pace to a point where I was virtually racing and I managed to get back alongside this random stranger who, let's face it, was probably about to feel very confused and threatened by my presence in her personal space.

I ignored the twinges of pain in my injured foot and kept surging on until a glance over my shoulder confirmed that I was strides ahead. What did I say earlier about ignoring pain, hey? Told you… Fickle!

Yay! I felt a little burst of joy. I'd passed her!

Then I felt a little pang of shame as I realised my whole effort was entirely pointless. It's not like we started at the same point or were heading for the same finish line. We weren't running the same distance or the same pace. Neither of us had any clue who the other person was and she probably hadn't even realised we were racing.

Unless…

Did she realise we were racing?

Is that why she passed me in the first place?

Did she actually start this race?

Perhaps I didn't need to feel the pangs of shame; I was simply competing in the race that she had initiated between us. And if so, I won!

Yes, I think I won.

I've convinced myself of my victory… Have I convinced you?

No?

OK – as much as I'm trying to justify it and appease my shame, it's most likely that she was unaware of any running rivalry between us that morning. Probably the only thing she was aware of was the feeling of uneasiness I left her with after encroaching on her personal space and muttering "In your faaaaace…" as I ran past.

The second time I glanced back, she was gone. I think she took a swift exit down a side path. Or possibly jumped in a sand dune to hide. Either way…

Actually, could she be the person who replied to my request above with:

- A scary, red-faced stranger who tried to race me while I was just out on a training run, minding my own business…

Chapter Thirteen
Real Life Top Tips

If you search the internet for running tips, you will get approximately 1,680,375,421. For anyone who, like me, can never read numbers past four digits, that's one billion, six hundred and eighty million, three hundred and seventy-five thousand, four hundred and twenty-one.

Don't quote me on that as it's only a rough count.

If after reading all those you find you still have unanswered questions, you can ask your running friends for their advice. You can expect to get approximately 2,710,428,197 top tips.

If after listening to all your running friends share their words of wisdom you still need support then a last resort is to refer to your non-running friends, who will happily dole out 9,100,873,127 facts about running because obviously they know best. Even if you don't resort to your non-running friends they will probably offer the advice unsolicited anyway.

When you factor in that roughly 95% of these billions of top tips are of absolutely no use whatsoever (again, don't quote me on the figure!) and almost every piece of advice is in direct conflict with another, what started out as a simple Google search to see if there was an ideal running buff for winter will leave you dazed and confused, wandering around the house muttering to yourself and contemplating your life choices (again!).

To help you in this running minefield, I've pulled together my favourite top tips from friends and family and compiled them into a handy list for future reference. You can decide which ones you take on board in your running but remember that I am not responsible for you – if any of the following cause you to have an epic running fail, that's on you.

You have been warned!

In no particular order, and with my own thoughts to follow where I have any:

- If you want to be a runner, you just have to run.
- Always dress for your second mile; it exists on an entirely different weather system to mile one.
- Join a running club.

I agree. There's not much more to be said on that!

- You can walk in your running shoes but you can't run in your walking shoes! Get the best pair you can afford that suit you and your running style, ability and routine. You can run without an expensive watch or fancy kit but decent running shoes are a must.
- Always, always, always warm up and cool down.

I am literally laughing out loud as I type this one out as I know a grand total of 1% of the running population will follow this advice, myself excluded!

- Factor in recovery weeks to your training plan;

don't just take them when you finally think you need them. It's too late by then. Your body needs regularly scheduled time to repair and gain strength between your runs.

- Your body is one moving part – don't neglect your core!

Again, I'm laughing out loud and shaking my head as I type. I do a Runner's Yoga YouTube video once every five to six months, if that counts.

- Leave your running comfort zone occasionally; it helps to keep apathy and boredom at bay.
- Face the traffic when you run.

This one is really important to me, especially with the increased number of electric cars on the road that are impossible to hear coming. I like to be able to see what is heading directly for me.

- Running should be enjoyable. If you're not enjoying some element of it and you actually hate every moment (as in genuinely hate the whole thing – not just that you hate the tough parts of a run but you love it after you've finished) then you have to ask yourself if it really is the hobby for you. Maybe try something else! Golf? Bingo? Knitting?
- Enjoy the easy runs and the social runs. Training and racing aren't everything.
- Run like there's a hot person in front of you and a creepy person behind you.

If you're following the hot person in front, are you their creepy person behind?

- Eat the right food.

Ha, yeah, OK! Good one!

- Always stay hydrated throughout the entirety of your running life.

I can say with complete certainty that I have never been fully hydrated a day in my life.

- Every runner should know their resting heart rate.

This didn't come with any further advice, so if you want to know more about why this is important, you will need to hit up your search engine of choice. All I can tell you from my own experience is that no matter how slow I try to run, my heart rate always suggests I am sprinting flat out, up a mountain, dragging a breeze block behind me. I was once doing heart-rate training at parkrun and had a hissy fit when I couldn't keep under the maximum heart rate designated by my coach. My gorgeous friend Verity breezed past me, coincidentally doing the same form of training in exactly the same heart-rate zone as I was meant to be, and she was having no trouble at all. I gave up and turned back after one lap, furious with the coach for setting such an unrealistic goal. It had nothing to do with my appalling fitness, obviously!

- Be realistic with your abilities – don't give yourself goals that are too far out of reach.

Another top tip that I fail to live by, even though I know it is very sensible. As I type, I am thinking about the marathon I just signed up for, taking place in five months. I'm currently running 12 miles a week recovering from my foot injury and I'm about to be fitted with some running orthotics that will take me back down to 30 minutes running, once a week, for the first month. I'm also writing 70,000+ words of a running book as well as working 36 hours, managing a home, learning French and looking after an aging relative. I also just joined Rock Choir to occupy another few hours of my rapidly declining free time. But yes, I still think I can train for and run a marathon in 150 days! The worst bit is, my so-called running friends are like, "Yeah, totally, that's so doable!"

Edit 1: the marathon is now 28 days away and I am currently huffing and puffing my way around a slightly painful 5k, once or twice a week.

Edit 2: the marathon was six months ago and I did not do it. I also did not finish this book on time. I did, however, master a few of the more important sentences in French: 'J'adore les croissants' (I love croissants) and 'Je cours lentement' (I run slowly).

- Concentrate. As much as it's nice to zone out, you have to take some responsibility for the other pedestrians, traffic and hazards you might come across.

And you don't want to miss out on great views and scenery. For years, I ran past a life-sized grizzly bear carved out of a tree and a life-sized wooden giraffe peeping over a fence without ever spotting them.

- You don't have to run in miles or kilometres just because everyone else does. It's totally OK to run in minutes and seconds if that is easier for you to manage.

- Trust the experts!

This is a good example of where it gets tricky with advice and top tips. Recently my very trusted podiatrist, who has helped me through a lot of issues, said I had a tight soleus that was causing me lots of problems. One day later, a sports therapist (not my usual one!) who has also helped me with lots of issues said my soleus was in great shape. I trust them both completely but as they were looking at the same leg, 24 hours apart, I must admit I was slightly confused!

- Learn from your mistakes.
- If part of you wants to go out and run but part of you thinks a run right now would be worse than taking a long hot bath in hell, go for a short walk instead but do it in your running kit. Once you are out, you might find the mood strikes and you do actually end up running. If not, just enjoy the walk and be pleased that you've still done some physical activity.

This one is my own top tip! Well, I suppose someone else may have said it before me, but I thought it up for myself not having read or heard it elsewhere, so I'm claiming it.

- Nip Guards and Body Glide are your two best running friends.

This one is from Stuart, who has returned home from many a rainy run with two trails of blood running down his T-shirt and the skin hanging off his thighs.

- Never trust a fart after mile one.

This one may also be from Stuart!

- Careful where you put your sunblock, as sweating will cause it to drip into your eyes.

This tip was given to me by a running friend but unfortunately I did not heed it myself and last week, in the middle of a four-day heatwave (It was hot. Maybe too hot!), I found myself mid-run with the most incredible stinging in my eyes. I genuinely thought I was going to go blind (I can be a bit dramatic, as you know).

- Start small on your foam roller; they are far more menacing than they look.

I can concur on this one! When I first shopped for a foam roller I made the assumption that the smooth, flat, shiny one would be no use at all and that if I was going to get maximum benefit from it, I needed the one with sinister-looking bumps (the ones that look like Toblerone pieces but less delicious). It was far too aggressive for what I needed and a complete waste of £25. I've discovered that you have to learn the foam roller; you can't really just climb on and roll, even though it sounds like you could. It takes quite a bit of practice, precision and tolerance before you progress from the basic smooth roller to the bumpier ones ('bumpy' is definitely the technical terminology used by foam roller experts).

- Relax. Running with clenched fists and hunched shoulders actually uses up energy that you could spend on your running instead.

Basically, chill out and go faster!

- If you don't stop to say hello to every dog on your run, you are not a runner!

Naturally! Or natch, as they say on social media. Stuart has never believed me when I've explained that 'natch' is well-used slang for the word 'naturally', so I am putting it in a book to prove him wrong!

Is that enough top tips for now? It feels like it should be enough to be getting on with. I certainly don't want to have to type out all ten billion tips that the internet and your friends and family have to share. If you do feel like you need more helpful advice, you might consider reading an actual running book, written by a running expert.

Chapter Fourteen
Real Life Running FAQs

There's been a lot of ground covered over the last thirteen chapters, so, to bring everything together in one handy, easy to read section near the end, I give you:

Real Life Running FAQs!

This chapter contains all (OK, not *ALL*) the questions likely to be asked by runners new and old alike (not old as in age, just old as in experience) and it's all gathered together in one chapter.

It can be used in a variety of ways.

The next time a non-runner asks you the same question for the hundredth time, e.g. "Doesn't it ruin your knees?" you can simply hand them this chapter.

Or, if you have a non-running friend who shows even the slightest bit of interest the next time you mention running, you can rapidly tear out the pages and thrust them in their face. They'll either be terrified or signed up to a race by that evening.

NB Please don't give them the whole book because, you know, sales figures!

Finally, if you're ever down in the dumps about your running and just want a laugh, or to remind yourself why we go on this absurd adventure, cast your eyes over the FAQs, which essentially provide a framework, albeit somewhat flimsy, for how to be a runner in real life.

In no particular order:

Q: Do I *need* any special kit for running?
A: No, just a pair of trainers and some comfortable fitness clothes.

Q: Will I *want* any special kit for running?
A: Yes. An expensive, high-spec, multi-function GPS running watch (replaced every Christmas and birthday), six pairs of advanced technology running shoes (a pair for road, a pair for trail, a pair for cross-country, a pair for fast running, a pair for slow running and a pair for special occasions), full-length leggings, cropped-length leggings, long shorts, short shorts, twin-layer shorts, a skort, 16 pairs of running socks (everyday run, training run, twin skin, ankle sock, compression, three-quarter-length, marathon and a variety of extra pairs to clog up your drawers), 10-15 technical vests, 50+ technical T-shirts (you will often get these for free at races but you will want to buy more nonetheless), a running club vest, a running club hoody, a running club sweatshirt, a running club pullover, a running club waterproof jacket, a running club soft shell jacket, a sun visor, a black running cap for winter, a white running cap for summer, a bobble hat, a beanie hat, a buff, a headband, a long-sleeved base layer, a short-sleeved base layer, three spiky balls of varying sizes, three resistance bands of various strengths, a heart-rate monitor, a single-bottle water

belt, a double-bottle water belt, a water hydration pack, a Freetrain, a pair of sunglasses (must be running branded and sports style), a clip-on waist purse, a flip-over waist belt, a flashing armband, a high-vis vest, two sweatbands (wrist and head), a head torch for night running, a sports bra (likely only to be replaced every five years), a pair of thick gloves, a pair of thin gloves and a pair of medium gloves.

Q: I only ever want to run 5k. Is that OK?
A: Yes – but see if you still feel the same after your first few 5ks, after which refer to the following sub-questions, as appropriate.

Q: I only ever want to run 10k. Is that OK?
A: Yes – but see if you still feel the same after your first few 10ks.

Q: I only ever want to run a half marathon. Is that OK?
A: Yes – but see if you still feel the same after your first few half marathons.

Q: I only ever want to run a marathon. Is that OK?
A: Yes – but see if you still feel the same after your first few marathons.

Q: Will other runners try and 'encourage' me to run longer distances than I think I would like?
A: Yes, they absolutely will. All the time. Incessantly.

Q: Can I politely decline?

A: You can try.

Q: How far should my first run be?

A: As far as you like or as far as you can manage. Don't forget that whatever distance you run, you have to run back. It's easy to get carried away on the first run. Perhaps plan an out-and-back route or a circular loop before you go, just to be safe.

Q: How much do races cost?

A: How much have you got?

Q: What is it like joining a running club?

A. Do you like to be surrounded by like-minded people who are as nuts as you are when it comes to running and will only ever want to talk about running, do running or talk about running a bit more? If not, definitely do not join a running club. However, if that does sound like you, find a club and sign up now (see below for how to find a club). If you look back at chapter one, you'll be reminded of why there is nothing to fear from joining a club.

Q: What does PB stand for?

A: Personal Best. Sometimes referred to as PR – Personal Record. You can have all sorts of PBs (or PRs): a distance PB, a race PB, a training PB, a post-injury PB, a parkrun PB, a Tuesday PB, a trail PB, a road PB, a yearly PB, a post-hangover PB... You can be as tenuous as you like with your PB categorisation.

Q: Will I really care about getting PBs?
A: Not at first. But later, yes. There's a good chance they will become the only thing you care about, even when you say you don't.

Q: Is running really bad for your knees?
A: Ask your non-running friend; they know the answer.

Q: I have a broken leg and my race is in two weeks. Will I be able to run it?
A: Please discuss this with your medical professional. Who should say no.

Q: Why is parkrun so popular?
A: It's wonderful. Next question.

Q: When will I be successful in the London Marathon ballot?
A: Peruse the comments section of London Marathon's last Facebook post and you will find a surprisingly high number of people who know all about organising world-famous marathons for 40,000 competitors, including a professional field. Any one of them will explain why you should be eligible for a place immediately.

Q: I have Achilles tendinopathy‡‡*. I stopped running for one day and did three of the five stretches that my sports therapist recommended but nothing has worked. Why?
A: Reread the question. Slowly.

Q: Where is the best location for a wild wee?
A: According to my expert friend Wendy, the best location for a wild wee is in a field of bluebells.

Q: How often is cake involved in running?
A: Always. If you run and there is no cake at the end, you have run with the wrong people. Find new running friends immediately. If you ran alone and there was no cake at the end, you have failed as a runner and a functioning human.

Q: Where can I get advice on local running clubs?
A: Google or your preferred search engine is a good place to start. A search for 'local running clubs' and your location should suffice. Another good way to scope out the local running scene is to spectate at a race (which you will probably have to find out about via Google or your preferred search engine. A search of 'local running races' and your location should suffice).

At local races, you'll see a lot of runners donning race vests from their respective running clubs and you

---

‡‡ Insert any running injury here

can make a note of the names and research them afterwards. Pick vests that come in the most flattering colours and styles.

Another good way to integrate into the scene and find a running club is to go to your local parkrun (www.parkrun.org.uk/events) and say to the very first person you find waiting in the start funnel, "Hi, I'm new." You'll be signed up to their running club by lunchtime. This one is a bit of a lottery, obviously; I hope you get someone nice!

Q: How do I find out about races?
A: See above!

Is that enough FAQs for now? It feels like it should be enough to be getting on with. I certainly don't want to have to type out ALL ten billion FAQs that runners might have. If you do feel like you have an unanswered question, you may consider reading an actual running book, written by a running expert.

NB If the last paragraph felt familiar, it's because it is almost word for word the same as the last paragraph of the previous chapter. I just copied it and changed the odd word. After fourteen chapters, I really am running out of things to say at this point!

Chapter Fifteen
Real Life Runners' Stories

When I started writing this book, I asked running friends and Instagram followers to share their stories with me via a questionnaire. I wanted to get some simple, genuine stories of how normal people got into running, why they do it and what they enjoy. Nothing glamorous; no sweeping declarations of undying love for the sport just to make it sound like the most amazing thing ever in order to sell the book. Just real, honest accounts that might resonate with some other runners and give a nod to our community spirit.

Here are a few of them.

Sam's Story

How did you get into running?
I met Dave and Angela, who are active members of the local running club, at a church group they lead. They began each group session with exercise. I knew they were runners and when I joined I made it clear I would only be walking and definitely not running, as that was not for me!

A couple of years later, inspired by a work

colleague (a non-runner) who had trained for and run the London Marathon for charity, I registered in secret for parkrun and went along to the War Memorial Park in Coventry one Saturday. I did not know if I could run even a hundred feet but I completed it in 43:30, surprising myself at how much of it I could run… Well, jog! That was over six and a half years ago!

What do you enjoy most about being a runner?
The simplicity of it. Also, being outside in the elements. Plus the social side too.

What injuries or awkward moments have you had?
I fell over on a run in an unfamiliar park, narrowly avoiding broken glass, and cut my knee and hand. It was all while I was doing a favour for my daughter and getting her car some new tyres fitted. I continued running back to the garage, where I went into their loo to clean myself up and ended up getting locked in. I had to shout for help, which made me cry. It was not my best impromptu run!

What's on your running bucket list?
To compete in the London Marathon – particularly now I have breast cancer – possibly raising funds for a charity supporting breast cancer sufferers.

What is your top tip for other runners?
Keep going if you enjoy it and don't beat yourself up over pace and time.

Nicola's Story

How did you get into running?

I've been running for almost two years now. When I first started out it was just me and my sister. We then joined a running group in Stratford, which helped us build our confidence with running and gave us some insight into different techniques and training classes to shake it up a bit. At first, I could only manage a Jeff; I loved being a Jeffer. With my asthma I found it hard to run a solid half mile without getting out of breath, so I began to work on how I ran. Everyone kept saying to breathe in through the nose and out through the mouth… Well, what an impossible task for an asthmatic! I found the more I tried to concentrate on breathing in that pattern, the more out of breath I became. I realised that the secrets to running a solid 5k without stopping for a breath are 1) keep to a pace I feel comfortable with, and 2) stop thinking about how I'm breathing and just let my body do what it's going to do. I can now run a distance up to a half marathon, but between 10k and 13.1 miles, I do like to be a Jeffer still.

What do you enjoy most about being a runner?

Running has given me a sense of relief, it helps me with my anxiety, it has improved my depression and, most of all, it's given me the ability to have a decent night's sleep.

Is there anything you don't enjoy about being a runner?
The actual running experience is more of a love/hate relationship: I love to sign up, I hate mass starts, I love it when I'm ready to go, I hate starting out and hitting a wall, I love it when I've got my pace finally under control, I hate it when I know how far I have left to run, I love it when the finish line is in sight and I can grab my medal! See what I mean? Love/hate! But, on a serious note, I do love to run; it's just overcoming those barriers that makes the entire run worth it in the end.

Prior to becoming a runner, were you aware of any myths or did you have any worries about running or joining a running club?
When I first joined a running club I was worried I wouldn't be fast enough. I always thought you had to run at a set minimum pace to be able to join the group. This isn't the case; everyone has their own pace and anyone is welcome to join. However, I did find with one club I would often be left far away at the back with no tail runner. Luckily, my sister would be ahead and would wait for me. I found this happened often and it made me think: "What's the point?"

So we left that club and decided to join a club called Fordy Runs. There was no local club and the majority of its members are all over the country, so we decided to start up a satellite group in Coventry and Warwickshire. The aim was that my sister would be run leader as she's quicker than me and I'd take the tail running. We wanted a group where pace doesn't matter; we want people to run however they feel comfortable and not worry they'll be left behind. So I always run at the back so that never happens to someone else like it did me. The group has come a long way and so have its members; we started with people who couldn't run more than a mile without stopping. They've overcome this and they can now run 5k without stopping, which is fantastic! Some of them are even attempting their first 10k with us shortly.

What was your first race?
An inflatable 5k was my very first attempt at a run and to be honest I think it was a great starting point. At this stage I still couldn't run a mile without Jeffing, so the inflatables were a welcome break in between. I really enjoyed the day; it made me feel like I was able to do more and I even signed up to more runs after this one. I think any run with an incentive is a good reason to run, right? Playing on inflatables, chocolate 5ks, colour runs, medals and T-shirts… What's not to like about races like this!

What is your greatest running achievement?
My greatest achievement is Canicrossing – it takes a lot to get into a flow/consistent pace with it and it's

very challenging. Everyone thinks it's easy with the dog pulling you, but that's not the case; it's more like "Can I keep up with this dog?" or, worse, "Will this dog ever stop?" and "Oh look, a bush – thanks for the diversion, Buddy, but a bit of warning would have been nice!"

It's great fun but you've first got to get used to it and know the habits and behaviours of the dog you're running with. My number one achievement is coming first in the novice class on my first race weekend. Granted, it was only between me and one other person rather than the usual 10 or 12 people, but it still made me proud.

What is your most embarrassing running moment of all time?
Wild weeing!

Originally it was my most embarrassing moment, but now it's just the norm! The first time I ever wild weed I was embarrassed, couldn't find a hedge I felt was concealing enough and had that moment of "Oh god, I can't pee whilst people are waiting!" and "People might see me, oh my!"

But no one batted an eye, no one cared, so after that I had no issue with it! Haha!

Have you ever fallen over or picked up an injury?
During the COVID-19 lockdown in May 2020, I decided to start running solo and get my fitness up rather than sitting around indoors not being able to do

anything or see anyone. I went for a run in the heatwave and although I felt like I was struggling a bit, I was going to push myself to go further. I got to a bridge, which I ran up, but two minutes later I was flat as a pancake sprawled out across the floor face first in front of the local pub. Luckily for me, pubs were closed and not many cars were on the road for anyone to see me and laugh. Even so, I felt like a right idiot and, quite frankly, the thought crossed my mind about not running anymore! I rang my mother to pick me up and I hobbled and cried my way towards home.

I got a card from my sister in the post (as I couldn't see or run with her during lockdown), which I've kept to this day. It says: "The one who falls and gets up is so much stronger than the ones who never fall. Keep going, Nicola, you're doing great" along with a nice, personalised message on the inside. This keeps me going and inspires me when I find it hard to get out and get motivated.

Have you ever seen anything odd on your run?
A running shoe… How is it possible for someone to lose a single shoe on a non-muddy run?! It still amazes me how they may have carried on without it.

Do you have a running pet peeve?
Runners that spit.

What's on your running bucket list?
My bucket list includes taking part in a Wolf Run, a

donut run, a wine run, complete a run in another country, take part in the Disneyworld Florida run (that one may never happen; have you seen the prices?!) and do a run in fancy dress. My running goals are to do a 5k in under 30 minutes (which I recently achieved) and run a 10k in less than an hour (which I am working on). My running dreams are that I'd like to have a try at a triathlon and attempt the Alpha Wolf – but let's not be too hasty!

Do you have any top tips for other runners?
Run at a pace that makes you feel comfortable, push yourself if you're up to it but most of all have fun. It's got to be enjoyable and beneficial to you so you want to keep on doing it. Find your reason and keep on going.

Louise's Story

How did you get into running?
I started running in January 2017. Well, I say running – I started Canicross, which is running with a dog (or dogs!). I have a lurcher called Chloe and at the time she was mental; walks were just not tiring her out and she was destroying my house! After lots of training and research, I decided she needed a job! I looked at agility classes but there were none around that fit around my stupid long hours and then someone

suggested Canicross. I Googled it and thought, "What?! You want me to run with my dog? R.U.N? Really?" There was a local group, so I decided I would have a go. We did about half a mile at the max – Chloe ran ahead like crazy and I tried to keep up… I thought I was going to die! She loved it though and did so well. She then slept most of the day and looked so happy.

So I signed us up for the following week. After a few weeks I too started to enjoy it as much as Chloe, so we purchased our own kit and started C25k (Couch to 5k) together. And that's where our journey started!

Four years later, we race most weekends during the Canicross season, which is September to March, and I now even run without her. We've also recently added a second lurcher to our family who I'm training up to run with us.

What do you enjoy most about being a runner?
Getting outdoors, exercising with my dog, and just ignoring everything going on in the world.

What was your first race? How did it go? How did you feel?
My first race was with Chloe in September 2017. I remember being super nervous and having about 10 wees beforehand! It was a novice race and due to the heat the route had been shortened; it was only about 2km but to me it felt like so much more at the time. I remember really trying and putting so much effort in and being so pleased when I finished and so pleased with how Chloe ran.

Did you make any 'rookie mistakes' when you first started running?

Not having the right shoes for trails and the organiser having to help me find some. Not knowing how to warm up properly and hurting myself.

What is your best running moment of all time? Or your greatest running achievement?

My greatest moment was doing the Longhorn 10km in 2019 with my sister. She did her furthest Canicross ever and she beat all her times. It was such a lovely run and route.

What is your worst running moment of all time?

My worst moment was out on a training run looking for a new 10km route for the Canicross Club. My friend climbed up a huge embankment as we had ended up stuck down the bottom of a disused railway. She let her dog off with us at the bottom as it was easier for her to call him and for him to find his own way to her. But her voice was thrown down the valley and the dog shot off the wrong way in a panic looking for her.

I quickly strapped my dog to a post and ran after him before he got too far away. Unfortunately, someone had dumped an old car chair with the rails attached. I saw the chair in the long grass but not the rails… I was just about to grab the dog's harness when I felt this immense pain in my shin. I grabbed the dog and looked down to find I had impaled my leg on the runners of the car chair. I made my way to the hospital and luckily I had missed the muscles and bone but it was really deep. It kept opening up and was so painful, I had to have three weeks off work.

What is the oddest thing you've seen on a run?
I once found myself being chased by sheep when out running with Chloe. I ended up picking her up and carrying her to get her out of the field quickly.

What's on your running bucket list?
I would love to eventually try and run a marathon! Also, I'd love to enter some races around Europe, maybe in Spain or France. Oh, and compete for Team GB in Canicross.

Do you have any top tips for other runners?
Make sure you always stretch, post-run. And keep well hydrated. Take a hydration pack if you need to, even if it's only a short run – don't be afraid of looking silly.

Sonia's Story

How did you get into running?
I've been running since January 2015. I tried to take up running a few times with friends/family in the mid-1990s and then again a couple of times in 2010 but I

only achieved any degree of success when I joined my teenage daughter on the NHS Couch to 5k. She listened to the app and I followed her. She's not a morning person, so there was very little conversation during our walking bits.

I'd already decided to join parkrun once I completed the C25k and a friend took me along with her. That's when I realised I had run for 30 minutes but never actually managed a full 5k! A year later, I joined Massey Ferguson Running Club and their RaceFit course and I haven't stopped running since; everything from 5ks to marathons.

What do you enjoy most about being a runner?
Finishing! No matter how hard a training run starts off or how tough a race gets, it always feels good at the end. Running with friends is brilliant because the miles fly by.

Did you have any worries about running?
So many non-runners say that running isn't good for your knees but all the articles I have read say it's great as a load-bearing exercise and for strengthening bones.

What was your first race?
My first race was the Massey Ferguson Running Club Easter 5 Miler. I hadn't done enough RaceFit homework so I was very stop-start throughout, with plenty of walking breaks, but the experience gave me

a baseline to improve upon.

Did you make any 'rookie mistakes' when you first started running?
See above! Another common rookie mistake in races is thinking it's impossible to catch the runner in front and forgetting that it is chip-timed. It's worth pushing that little bit more because, even if you don't overtake them, you might still have a faster time if they started before you. Always try to close that gap!

What is your best running moment of all time?
My first marathon – Virgin Money London Marathon 2018 and the hottest one in history. Spotting various family and clubmates in the crowds en route was the best feeling ever. Likewise, the support and encouragement from complete strangers was unbelievable. My two youngest daughters were watching the race on television and recorded their reaction at the moment I crossed the finish line – that was magic! The BBC race coverage literally finished a minute after I crossed the line!

Have you ever had a 'kit mishap'?
No, but I often dream about having the wrong kit on when running a race. How do you interpret that?

Have you ever seen anything odd on your run?
Only a muntjac deer leaping across the road within inches of me.

What's on your running bucket list?

The simple one I want to do is the Chester Triple, which is a 10k in March, a half marathon in May, and a marathon in October. Unfortunately, COVID-19 got in the way but I'll do it one year. I'd also like to run in some events overseas but I haven't worked out which ones yet!

Have you had any good celebrity spots during a race?

The newsreader Sophie Raworth at Fulham Palace parkrun in February 2020. I can't tell you what she was like, other than she was so fast I didn't see her finish.

What do your family think of your running activities?

They are proud of my progress over the years but I bore them silly with running stories because they aren't runners themselves!

Do you have any top tips for other runners?

If you're following a training plan, don't overtrain as you might get an overuse injury. And don't beat yourself up if life gets in the way and you have to skip a training run. If you enjoy running and need running buddies, join a friendly running club. There are always other runners that will give you advice and encouragement and you will find opportunities to give something back too.

Lia's Story

How did you get into running?

I started running in high school in 2007. My mom had been into running as long as I could remember, so I figured I would try it out. I did my first half marathon with a long training run of 5 miles because my boyfriend at the time thought we could do it. I actually trained more than him if that's even possible! Dumb! I couldn't walk; it was terrible! But I kept going and started running properly with my mom and eventually I got hooked.

I've now done 22 half marathons and 11 full marathons. I've done New York Marathon, Las Vegas, the Dopey Challenge, Washington, Victoria, and many others in between. My mom has been my BIGGEST supporter and we have often planned running vacations together.

Since I had kids we've put the running trips on hold and I don't know if she would ever do another marathon herself, but she is definitely encouraging and I know she will help me any way possible so I can keep running.

What do you enjoy most about being a runner?

The time to myself and setting new goals to work towards. I need something to work towards and strive for, else I just do the same old thing and get bored too easily. I like pushing myself and seeing what I am capable of.

Is there anything you don't enjoy about being a runner?
Blisters and black toenails!

What was your first race?
WPS (Winnipeg Police Service) half marathon in 2010. It was awful. It rained sideways and was so windy and cold. I couldn't move for, like, five days. I said I was never going to do it again but I did, of course!

What is your best running moment of all time?
I have three!
1) I think finishing a race feeling good and not defeated or depleted. I had someone tell me at mile 22 of a marathon that I looked way too good at that point in the race. That boosted my confidence way up! That told me I raced a smart race and trained smart.
2) Going to Blowing Rock, North Carolina for a running camp. It was so much fun! It was four days of just learning about running.
3) Taking my marathon coaching certification. It has helped me a lot in my own running and I am sharing my knowledge with other people, which I totally enjoy! Maybe one day I'll do something more with it but for now I'm enjoying sharing the information with those who ask.

What is your worst running moment?
I tripped on a curb on the sidewalk at mile 17 of a race and landed on my chin. Blood everywhere! I still

finished though and even PR'd!

What should you never say to a runner?
1) Running is bad for your knees.
2) I signed up for my first 5k marathon.
3) I can't run. I hate it.

What do your family think of your running activities?
They don't think twice about it. It's part of my life. My daughter loves to come in the stroller and the other day grabbed my running shoes, put them on and said, "I'm going to run."

Do you have any top tips for other runners?
Don't worry about pace or other people's perception of your running. Just run.

Simone's Story

Simone is my sister. She is not currently, nor has she ever been a runner, to my knowledge, so I was surprised to receive a notification telling me she'd offered her running story to share with us. Pleasantly surprised, I made a cup of tea, grabbed a couple of custard creams (Stuart's pre-race breakfast of choice!) and sat down on the sofa to leisurely read through her story. This is what she wrote, verbatim…
I barely had time to eat one custard cream!

I have something but it would be no good for your book LOL because there was not one bit of running going on with either Chad or me… There wasn't even a slight jog here or there. It was barely a walk really, with frequent stops to resume normal breathing, ward off the vomiting and nausea and mop up the sweat. And trust me, this was not like a light 'produce mist' kind of sweat, we were literally dripping! Had we been actually somewhat running, we would have been a bio-hazard risk, I kid you not!

Chad talked me into this race as it was for charity and it was the beginning of May. It would be nice cool weather, he said; it would be fun, he said…

Turns out we had an unprecedented heatwave for May that day plus, apart from the start and finish lines, the entire route was all uphill. Even the dog got a nosebleed! We both thought we were going to die in the middle of City Park. And it was so humiliating, with all the young mums flying past us with their jogging strollers, old folks leaving us in their wake, kids laughing at us as they whizzed past on their bikes. I wanted nothing more than to kick them off the darn things! There are honestly no words to express the horror, seriously!

I do remember about a third of the way through thinking to myself that actually Chad isn't that great and I started to become quite comfortable with the thought of breaking up with him.

Never again, and as it turns out we could have just donated the entry fee – there was no need to participate at all. And Chad knew that! The whole thing was just tragic!

We even had to buy the race T-shirts… The itchy and uncomfortable T-shirts. I swear they were made out of potato sacks. The material is so tough it practically stands up on its own! LOL!

I don't think Simone is going to be joining a running club any time soon, is she? However, being the eternal optimist that I mentioned I am in Chapter One, and thinking that we might one day enjoy runs together, I purposely chose Simone's story as the very last words in this book (well, apart from 'The End'), so that when she reads it, looking to see if her story made the cut, she will have to read everything else beforehand and may find herself warming to the idea of running.

I doubt it – but you never know!

THE END

Printed in Great Britain
by Amazon